STUTTERING

Integrating Theory and Practice

Edited by

Jarg B. Bergold, Berlin
Niels Birbaumer, Tübingen
Irmella Florin, Tübingen
Dieter Kallinke, Heidelberg
Dietmar Schulte, Bochum
Wolfgang Tunner, München

STUTTERING

Integrating Theory and Practice

Peter A. Fiedler
Renate Standop

Translated by

S. Richard Silverman

from
STOTTERN
Wege zu einer integrativen
Theorie und Behandlung
Copyright © Urban & Schwarzenberg 1978

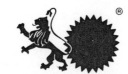

AN ASPEN PUBLICATION®
Aspen Systems Corporation
Rockville, Maryland
London
1983

Library of Congress Cataloging in Publication Data

Fiedler, Peter A., 1945-
Stuttering: integrating theory and practice.

Translation of: Stottern.
Bibliography: p. 189
Includes index.
1. Stuttering.   I. Standop, Renate.   II. Title.
RC424.F5313   1982   616.85′54   82-13818
ISBN: 0-89443-665-1

Publisher: John Marozsan
Editorial Director: R. Curtis Whitesel
Managing Editor: Margot Raphael
Editorial Services: Jane Coyle
Printing and Manufacturing: Debbie Collins

Copyright © 1983 by Aspen Systems Corporation

Library of Congress Catalog Card Number: 82-13818
ISBN: 0-89443-665-1

Printed in the United States of America

1   2   3   4   5

Table of Contents

Foreword ix

PART I—IDENTIFICATION, ORIGIN, AND MAINTENANCE OF
    STUTTERING 1

Chapter 1—Identification of Stuttering 3

       Introduction 3
       Basic Symptomatology 4
       What Stuttering Is Not 6
       Observable Patterns 7
       Responsibility of Stutterers for Communication 10
       Effects of Competing Stimulation and Activity 11
       Prevalence and Extent of Stuttering 12
       Summary 13

Chapter 2—Origin of Stuttering: Genetic and
       Somatic Hypotheses 15

       Introduction 15
       The Onset of Stuttering 15
       The Course of Early Childhood Stuttering 17
       Sex-Specific Distribution of Stuttering 20
       Familial Occurrence of Stuttering 21
       Organic Causes 22
       Summary 34

Chapter 3—Development and Maintenance of Stuttering:
       Psychological Research and Interpretation 37

204520

Introduction 37
Stuttering as Operant Behavior 38
Emotional Agitation and Stuttering 40
Stuttering as a Consequence of Diagnosis 42
Digression: Stuttering as Social Behavior 43
Cognitive-Social Aspects of Stuttering 46
Neuropsychological Aspects of Conflict 48
The Origin of Conflict and Development
    of Stuttering 49
The Social Role of the Stutterer and Its Predisposition
    to Conflict 51
Summary 52

Chapter 4—The Search for Integration: Stuttering as a
            Neuropsychological Phenomenon 55

Introduction 55
A Neuropsychological Model of the Origin and
    Maintenance of Stuttering 56
Interferences with Auditory Feedback and "Normal"
    Speech Disturbance 56
Developmental Stuttering 58
Retention of Auditory Speech Control and
    Symptomatic Stuttering 59
Speech Training and Symptomatic Stuttering 60
Heredity and Stuttering 61
The Maintenance of Stuttering and Subjectively
    Experienced Responsibility for Communication 62
External Control and Failure-Free Speech 63
A Paradox: Stuttering and the Subjective Effort To
    Improve Speech 64
Cognitive-Social Determinants of Stuttering 66
Summary 67

PART II—DIAGNOSIS AND THERAPY FOR STUTTERING 69

Chapter 5—A Diagnostic Schema for Preparation of Therapeutic
            Measures for the Treatment of Stuttering 71

Introduction 71
1. Description of the Speech Disorder 73
2. Description of Social Difficulties and Additional
    Conspicuous Behaviors 85

3. Differential Diagnosis of the Boundaries of the
   Speech Disorder 87
4. Analysis of Conditions 89
5. General Considerations in Preparing Therapeutic
   Measures 96

Chapter 6—Management of the Speech Disorder **99**

Introduction 99
Systematic Training in New Speech Habits 101
Fundamental Alteration of Speech Habits 119
Summary 123

**Chapter 7—Measures Preceding and Accompanying Treatment of
the Speech Disorder** **125**

Introduction 125
Training for Symptom Awareness
   (Self-Observation) 125
Sound and Video Recordings in Speech Therapy 127
Control of Breathing 131
Relaxation Techniques 132
Drugs and Speech Therapy 134
Summary 135

Chapter 8—Self-Control and Self-Modification of Stuttering **137**

Introduction 137
Therapist and Client 138
Implementation and Testing of Self-Modification 144
Summary 148

Chapter 9—Treatment of Social Disorders **149**

Introduction 149
General Requirements for Positive Transfer 150
Constructing Hierarchies of Situations Marked by
   Anxiety 151
Role Playing 151
Transfer of Training 157
The Role of Caretakers in Therapy 157
Summary 159

Chapter 10—Combination of Speech and Social Therapeutic Measures in the Treatment of Stuttering **161**

Introduction 161
Early Identification of Stuttering 162
Early Treatment of Childhood Stuttering 163
The Treatment of Stuttering in Older Children and
    Youths 166
Sequence of Therapeutic Steps 166
Combined Methods 169
Multidimensional Therapeutic Approaches 169
Integrative Behavior Therapy for Stuttering 171
Resocialization as a Concern of Behavior Therapy 175
The Function of Dialogue in the Treatment of
    Stuttering 176
Summary 178

Chapter 11—Results of Therapy and Prognosis **179**

Introduction 179
Measurement of Outcomes of Treatment 179
Relapse and Repetition of Therapeutic Experience 183
Causes of Relapse and Implications for Therapy 184

References **189**

Index **207**

Foreword

Despite the steadily increasing accumulation of knowledge about the origins and varying conditions of stuttering, the results of therapy particularly with regard to long-term effects have been disappointing until now. We therefore think it is well-advised to compare the manifold theoretical assessments and interpretations of causes and development of speech disorders and to examine the actual results of research directly. Moreover, we think it would be productive to present comprehensively in one volume the differing approaches to the management of stuttering that are currently employed in therapeutic practice and to compare them with one another.

Accordingly, this monograph is organized into two parts. Part I deals with the identification of the speech disorder "stuttering" (Chapter 1) as well as exposition of the various hypotheses concerning the origin and maintenance of stuttering (Chapters 2 and 3). We would like to show that despite variations in stated interpretations, there are many common elements and overlappings as well as structural similarities that we think constitute an appropriate basis for attempting theoretical integration. From the neuropsychological point of view which we present, the subjective experience of responsibility for communication on the part of the stutterer is the central connecting link between the somatic and the psychological determinants of stuttering. We believe that the propositions we shall explore represent a fruitful area for further research.

Part II works up systematically the continually growing "assortment" of therapeutic techniques (especially the management of difficulties of speech). We shall augment this exposition with the results of our practical work growing out of substantially controlled individual case studies carried out in the context of research projects at the Psychological Institute of the Westf, Wilhelms University in Münster. By means of the "diagnostic scheme for preparation of therapeutic measures" in Chapter 5 we hope to facilitate diagnostic preliminary work on which therapeutic intervention in practical cases is based. In Chapters 6 to 9 various approaches to management of stuttering are presented. In so doing our guide has been to describe therapeutic methods as clearly as possible in order to provide specific suggestions and tangible assistance in therapeutic practice. Nevertheless, we shall stress the point that therapy for stuttering is not confined to management of the speech disorder exclusively. Rather, and just as important, the therapist needs to establish broadened social competence of the client as an objective of his or her management along with the practice of those skills (especially cognitive) that will enable the client to achieve long-range self-control and self-modification of stuttering. The two concluding chapters address salient considerations concerning general design of therapy. Differentiation of management of children, adolescents, and adults will be discussed in Chapter 10. Pointers to accomplish positive transfer based on current findings will be summarized in Chapter 11.

Stuttering: Integrating Theory and Practice is addressed especially to psychologists, physicians, educators, rehabilitative and special educators, social workers, and others who are entrusted with the management and care of speech-handicapped persons.

We would like to thank the editors of the monograph series, especially Herr Prof. Dr. Dietmar Schulte, for including our monograph in the series. Thanks are also due those colleagues whose discussion and collaboration were helpful from the beginning of the undertaking, especially Dipl.-Psych. Hans-Joachim Hofmann, Dipl.-Psych. Horst Oertle, Dipl.-Psych. Roswitha Reincke, Dipl.-Psych. Bernd Schmidt, and Dipl.-Psych. Dr. Herwig Widlak.

Munster, 1978   PETER A. FIEDLER
                                                     RENATE STANDOP

Part I

Identification, Origin, and Maintenance of Stuttering

Chapter 1

Identification of Stuttering

INTRODUCTION

Despite a great deal of effort to come closer to understanding the theoretical and practical bases of the problem of stuttering, we are still very much in the dark about its causes. The feasibility of management of stuttering and the conditions under which it operates are so varied that it is not possible at this time to offer a uniform diagnostic-therapeutic approach. However, the clinical phenomena of stuttering are widely known and are amply described and classified (Heese, 1967; Arnold, 1970a; Sheehan, 1970; Böhme, 1977; to name only a few).

In the area of speech, especially in the medical literature, there are several synonyms in German for "stuttering": in common use are such terms as *balbuties* and *dysphemie,* in less common use, *spasmophemie* and *laloneurosa;* also in very early work the obsolete term *psellismus* occurs. In Anglo-American work *Stottern* is termed *stuttering* and, now and then, *stammering.* The German as well as the Anglo-American terminology for the particular phenomena and differentiations of stuttering is not at all uniform. Nevertheless, in recent years, particularly in clinical psychology, there appears to be evidence pointing to the development of a standard terminology. This, too, is one of the purposes of this introductory chapter, in which we introduce into the German speech context original, useful terminology related to the identification of observable distinctive features of stuttering.

Unfortunately, many speech experts disagree as to when to label a person a stutterer (Johnson, 1956a). However, there is generally wide agreement on the symptomatology of adult stutterers. Stuttering is a frequent, conspicuous interruption in speech fluency. It is characterized by an abrupt block before a word, a syllable, or a phoneme. Delays, prolonging and shortening the production of single sounds, as well as repetition of words and parts of sentences occur. Unnecessary sounds are also inserted. This deviant speech is frequently accompanied by abnormal breathing and by inappropriate coordination of involved muscle groups: lasting for seconds, tense opening of the mouth or pressing together of the lips, teeth grinding on one another, clearly audible strokes of the glottis, thrusting, jerky movement of the tongue during pauses in speech, gasping inspiration during speech coinciding with the stuttering.

BASIC SYMPTOMATOLOGY

Interruptions in speech fluency are conventionally labeled either tonic or clonic stuttering.

Tonic stuttering is characterized by relatively prolonged tension of the speech musculature. This often leads to a silent straining that precedes the beginning or continuation of a word (for example: ". . . [pause]" or "poli . . . tics"). These tensions persist for a comparatively long time and are relieved only after great effort. Occasionally, clearly audible glottal strokes are manifest (a "rattling" soft noise produced by the impact on one another of the vocal bands).

Clonic stuttering is characterized by shorter contractions of the speech musculature that rapidly follow one another. Typically, it is like a "rat tat tat" repetition of sounds, syllables, or words so that definitive articulation results in prolongation of words (for example: "c-c-c-come" or "tow-t-t-t-el").

These two forms can occur separately or in combination. If one of the two so-called tensing conditions predominates we speak of clonic-tonic or tonic-clonic stuttering. Occasionally, there are references in the literature to frequent periods of remission of the disturbance that may range from clonic to clonic-tonic to tonic stuttering symptoms (Berendes & Schilling, 1962).

In English language studies explicit distinction between these two kinds of symptom classification is made only rarely. Moreover, when it does happen the use of terms is not uniform. Thus, Case (1960) labels clonic symptoms as *stuttering,* and tonic ones as *speech block.* But English language usage also permits clonic symptoms to be identified as *stammering* and tonic ones as *stuttering* (see Jussen, 1964, p. 166). According to Lehner (1960), the concept of speech block is conventionally reserved for more severe forms of the disorder; he objects to the synonymous use of the labels *stuttering* and *speech block.* Variation in the use of language makes comparison of investigations difficult, especially in experiments or accounts of therapy in which stuttering is not described operationally.

Many of the described symptoms also occur in the speech of normal-speaking persons. Stutterers, however, repeat parts of words approximately ten times more frequently than nonstutterers and whole words and parts of sentences three times more often. Stutterers produce incomplete sentences four times more frequently than normal talkers and terminate much more frequently in the middle of a word (Johnson, 1961). But Johnson (1967) also observed considerable speech disfluencies in some people who nevertheless were not labeled as stutterers and who did not consider themselves stutterers. Thus, for example, insertions such as "ah" or "um" that interrupt sentences, as well as word and sentence delays, occur as frequently with nonstutterers as with stutterers.

Accompanying Symptoms of Stuttering

An array of *conspicuous movements*, also called parakinesis (Arnold, 1970b; Heese, 1967), can accompany stuttering. Involved are bizarre movements of the muscles of the face and neck, of the extremities, or of the whole body, which are executed simultaneously with speech. Phenomenologically, they remind one somewhat of tics. Movements occur in varying manner and degree. Originally thought to assist the stutterer to overcome speech block more rapidly, they appear to have established themselves in the course of time as ineffective accompanying symptoms and come to affect nonverbal means of expression such as mimicking and gesture adversely. *Mimicking* is especially impaired by tonic symptoms. During the blockage of speech, spasmlike movements of the lips, tongue, or in the region of the eyes often occur. The stutterer frequently avoids direct eye contact. Calavrezo (1965) has called attention to the absence of *gesture* and *gesticulation*. In their place there are activities like finger snapping, beating the hand on the upper thigh, and the like. Often the body assumes a stiffened posture, for instance, by tense clinging to the back of a chair.

Flicklaute ("patching" sounds) or *Flickwörter* ("patching" words), also called *Embolophonien* or *Embolophrasien* (Heese, 1967), as, for example, "hmmm," "at any rate," "so to speak," etc., or other sounds inserted by stutterers more frequently than by normal speakers are likewise said to facilitate fluent speech. Furthermore, the fear of particular sounds or words that experience has marked as particularly vulnerable can give rise to alteration of choice of words or sentence construction. How important this is for the observer may depend, of course, on the size of the vocabulary on which the stutterer can draw.

There are additional rather prominent standard strategies that are also thought to contribute assistance and relief in overcoming blocks and hesitations during the moment of stuttering. Among these is a so-called *starter* (Widlak, 1977). Starters are parts of words or words or expressions that by and large can be produced failure free and are easy for the stutterer to say. They often serve as regular starting aids for articulation of difficult words and beginning of words. Starters are inserted especially at the time when the stutterer is impelled to speak by the press of the situation (for example, "Actually I have always been of the opinion that . . . ." or "If I must say . . . ."). One of the most renowned starters was used by Winston Churchill, who in adulthood used it to control his stuttering successfully. He inserted a long "hm" before the beginning of several of his sentences. Thus, for example, "Hmmmmmmm England will never surrender" was heard in a radio speech during World War II (cited by Schwartz, 1977).

For purposes similar to the starter, symptomatic stop-go mechanisms are inserted during recovery. These are reinserted by the stutterer immediately after cessation of blocks and at the beginning of articulation or by using entirely new words. These *rebounds* (called *recoil behavior* by Van Riper, 1971) can occur several times successively and, to some extent, with great rapidity.

Finally, breathing, that is, the holding of the breath, can be controlled in such a manner as to increase the probability of failure-free articulation. In doing this the stutterer can employ an array of methods of inspiration and expiration. Not infrequently *inspirational speech* is observed in which whole sentences are produced rapidly and correctly with inspiration though with conspicuously altered pitch, more like "breathing from within." Equally striking is *speaking with residual* air. Volumes of residual air in the lungs are used to speak longer constructions and sentences rapidly and correctly. Furthermore, Schilling (1965) describes a so-called *paradoxen Atemtyp* (paradoxical breathing type), by which he means "drawing in the abdominal wall with inspiration and raising and arching it with expiration" (p. 386).

All of these accompanying symptoms can appear more or less automatically. They generally resist change, depending on their nature and the duration of their development.

WHAT STUTTERING IS NOT

Stuttering needs to be distinguished from *Stammeln* (stammering) and *Poltern,* abnormally rapid speech (cluttering). *Stammering* is a defect in articulation. Particular sounds or combinations of sounds are incorrectly formed and are either omitted, substituted for, or imprecisely formed

(Berendes & Schilling, 1962). Speech should first be labeled *disordered,* when mistakes in production do not disappear in the course of speech development and when the period of physiological stammering common to most children persists beyond that time. *Cluttering* (also called *Tachyphemia*) identifies an abnormally rapid manner of speech combined with unintelligibility (Wallrabenstein, 1963). Cluttering is frequently confused with stuttering. The clutterer also repeats sounds, syllables, and words several times one after another. Or he or she blocks in the middle of a sentence. However, in cluttered speech the tensing of the speech musculature typical of stuttering is not present. Cluttering can occur along with stuttering. This makes differential diagnosis difficult. Occasionally, the opinion has been advanced that in some cases cluttering can lead to stuttering (Schmidt, 1969; Arnold, 1970a).

This distinction is found predominantly in the work of authors writing in the German language. In the Anglo-American speech field there is unmistakable disagreement about the need for differential diagnosis. Yates (1970) considers it of no use and not worthy of further attention. However, Beech and Fransella (1971) as well as Johnson (1967) advocate a distinction between stuttering and cluttering in order to facilitate a better comparison among results of research. This need is further emphasized in such problems as the relation between varied favorable prognoses and the perception of the disorder by the affected individual (see Chapters 5 and 11). In general we do not find a distinction in the English language between stuttering and stammering; they are frequently used synonymously.

Finally, stuttering needs to be distinguished from *speech disfluencies* that occur in the course of speech development in children. These, of course, are evident in the repetition of sounds, syllables, and words, which is normal for children between the ages of two and five. Thus, almost every child goes through a more or less conspicuous phase of *physiological stuttering,* to which we shall return in more detail later (Chapter 2 and Chapter 4).

OBSERVABLE PATTERNS

Particularly characteristic of stuttering is the variation of symptom frequency and severity under differing conditions. This leads to certain patterns that are important for the identification of stuttering. Among these patterns or regularities, abundantly reported in several studies, are those subsumed under the terms *consistency effect* and *adaptation effect.*

Consistency of Stuttering

The *consistency effect* refers to the tendency of a stutterer in repeated reading of the same text to stutter most frequently at the same place (Johnson, 1956b). Particular proximate sounds and words seem to have a persistent environmental influence on the tendency (Fierman, 1956). The portion of words stuttered on repeated readings of the text is approximately two-thirds of that stuttered on the first reading. This relation also holds for subsequent readings. Moreover, the consistency effect persists even after an interval of weeks between readings (Tate & Cullinan, 1962). Measurements of the consistency effect and severity of stuttering appear to be correlated (Shulman, 1956).

One explanation of the consistency effect is suggested by the possibility that the stutterer appraises the word to be spoken and therefore expects to stutter more or less severely. In this connection the terms *anticipatory effect* or *anticipatory phenomenon* are mentioned (Tunner, 1974). Stutterers can predict with great accuracy the words on which they will stutter. And when the same appraisal criteria are used by the stutterer as the basis for rating the severity of stuttering then the probability of stuttering on these words is greater than on others (Brown, 1945; Beech & Fransella, 1971).

Observations and analyses of consistency in stuttering suggest the following recurring interrelations among its various characteristics (Quarrington, 1956; Taylor, 1966; Heese, 1967):

- Stuttering on the first word or first words of sentences is observed more frequently than on words within sentences. Hence, initial sounds are stuttered more frequently than other sounds.
- Stuttering on long words is more likely than on short ones.
- Symptoms appear largely with grammatically significant words like substantives, adjectives, verbs, or adverbs.
- Stutterers experience greater difficulty in the production of consonants than of vowels and therefore anticipate more likely blocking on them; this is especially the case with initial consonants.

There is, to be sure, pure *vowel stuttering*. It is rather rare and hardly noticeable. Tessenow (1958) suggests that this is due to the fact that by and large most words begin with consonants and vowels within words hardly require any effort. A relation between the difficulty with particular sounds and their degree of phonetic-physiological difficulty is unlikely.

The stutterer can produce all the necessary sounds adequately (Brutten & Shoemaker, 1967).

Distinctive specifiable conditions that correspond to the implicit appraisal criteria assumed by Brown (1945) are noted. According to him stutterers attach significance and weight to such appraisals. They depend on the number of the aforesaid features a word contains. These assumptions are supported by the experimental results of Oxtoby (1956), who found that the frequency with which the same word was always stuttered was proportional to the number of the above-mentioned features that it contained. This experiment yielded an additional interesting result related to the consistency effect, namely, the influence of varying instructions on the frequency of stuttering. The greatest consistency occurred with the instruction to the stutterer to avoid stuttering. The least consistency occurred with the instruction to substitute "normal speech" for stuttering after gentle repetition of the first sound or the first syllable of a word.

Adaptation in Stuttering

The *adaptation effect* refers to a decrease in the frequency of stuttering with repeated readings at a particular place in a text (Johnson, 1956a). Review of research suggests an asymptotic adaptation curve. In most experiments adaptation was studied with reading and not with spontaneous speech. Obviously, reading could be controlled more easily. Generally in these cases a short text was read loudly five times in succession with brief pauses between renditions. In experiments of this type, frequency of stuttering was reduced about 50%. However, when the material of the text was changed in successive readings, the reduction was between 10 and 20% (Golub, 1956). The length of the text (at least in passages of 200, 500, and 1,000 words) had no significant effect on the amount of adaptation. On the other hand, the degree of adaptation was increased the shorter the interval between single readings (Shulman, 1956).

In addition to the nature of the material and the magnitude of the intervals between readings, the particular conditions associated with the readings had a significant influence on the effect. Van Riper and Hull (1956) emphasize the influence on adaptation of *environmental* factors. In their investigation they showed that experimentally determined adaptation levels could *not* be sustained under varying situational conditions (microphone and speaking in public). It is interesting to note here that the increase in symptoms was strongly proportional to the difficulty of the situation as perceived by the stutterer. A particularly intense increase in symptoms, to be sure, dependent on the severity of the stuttering, occurred in those people who had not yet come to terms with their symptoms. Although in another context, Heese (1967) observed that there is an improvement in the disorder when a "definite reconciliation with the stress" occurs (p. 21). Finally, in additional experiments the influence of the presence of people during the adaptation sessions was investigated. The results are indeed inconsistent (Beech & Fransella, 1971). This may be related to differing experimental procedures, for example, variation in kinds of reading material, steady improvement, or static level of listener judgments.

Despite the abundance of investigations of the adaptation effect, unequivocal use of the effect for treatment and prognoses has not been successful. And a definitive theoretical clarification is still not available. Yet there are interesting supplementary findings that are worthy of note here. Severe stutterers adapt less than moderate stutterers (Shulman, 1956). Severe and moderate stutterers differ both in the course and rapidity of adaptation (Van Riper & Hull, 1956). Moreover, age of the subjects plays a part and there is no transfer of the effect from reading to spontaneous speech (Harris, 1942). It has also been shown that the frequency of stuttering associated with adaptation reverts to the initial level. This has been called *spontaneous recovery* in stuttering (Johnson, 1956b).

RESPONSIBILITY OF STUTTERERS FOR COMMUNICATION

For most stutterers reading aloud is less disturbing than free speech. Hennig (1959) states that this definitely holds for children so long as the text is not exciting. This can occur, for example, when the text is in a foreign language and there is fear of making a mistake in speaking. In general, stuttering confined exclusively to reading occurs rarely (Arnold, 1970b). Performance in reading is especially more difficult if expectancy anxiety about particular sounds prevails. With predetermined texts it is not possible to avoid anticipated difficulties by altering the choice of words.

There are a number of situations in which a considerable decrease in symptoms or even their complete absence can be observed. Among these are speaking nonsense material and single words, counting and spelling, as well as singing and choral speaking. Stutterers experience hardly any difficulty in talking to themselves or in expressing themselves with children and animals. It is relatively easy for the stutterer to imitate or to repeat the speech of another person (Bloodstein, 1949).

In all of these conditions the importance to the talker of speech as a means of communication (we call this the *subjective experience of responsibility for communication*) is diminished. Normally, frequency of stuttering increases with the perceived importance or difficulty of the circumstances in which the stutterer intends to speak. Thus, there is an increase when in conversation with authorities or with larger numbers of listeners. Another example is the special difficulty on the telephone. Just the ring of the telephone gives rise to an attack in the middle of saying something. As many studies report, stuttering becomes more intense the more stutterers withdraw from a situation in which, up to a point, they had learned to control their speech, that is, when the number of strange and unfamiliar characteristics of a situation increases (Heese, 1967; Wendlandt, 1972).

In cluttering, in contrast to stuttering, there is usually a decrease in symptom severity when "good speech" is attained. Speech disfluencies of a clutterer appear more severe, for example, in exchanges with familiar persons compared with superiors (Arnold, 1970a).

The significance of responsibility for communication for the stutterer related to the onset and severity of symptoms obviously is important, just as the significance of the actual desire and need to speak is part of the stutterer's cognitive set, that is, whether a situation is judged to be somewhat easy or tough, familiar or unfamiliar, important or unimportant. Bloodstein (1949) suggests that the onset of stuttering is less likely if the stutterer anticipates an agreeable rather than an amused or impatient reaction from the listener. Generally crucial is the impression and the expectation of stutterers that they will be accepted by their interlocutors and that there will be less conspicuous attention to their speech disorder by others. This is often the case when family or friends are the listeners. Many stutterers, including children, have a minimum of difficulty when they are with such groups of people. This leads to an improvement in the responsibility for communication and often results in a substantial decrease in symptoms. Speech is usually also easier with socially or intellectually inferior persons. This particular status ensures security and relieves stutterers of the need to make a good impression on the listener (Bloodstein, 1949). Alone and then after acclimatization to provocative situations, the stutterer shows considerable improvement in speech difficulty, even if complete symptom-free speech is seldom achieved.

EFFECTS OF COMPETING STIMULATION AND ACTIVITY

A variety of *motor activities* (for example, finger snapping and foot stamping), which frequently become symptoms, are used as quickly as possible by many stutterers to overcome a speech block. They are said to facilitate the production of words and thus improve speech fluency. There is a large array of additional activities reported that, when instituted along with stuttering, similarly reduce symptoms, such as piano playing, athletic activity, walking, dancing, and writing. Additional ones that deviate from

normal patterns of speech are frequently suitable for reducing or completely eliminating stuttering. Bloodstein (1949) mentions a number of such
possibilities: whispering, speaking in a higher pitch, exaggerated articulation, imitation of dialect, many people speaking at once, and singing in
a choir. The singing of stutterers is disturbed only rarely.

The effect of stronger or abnormal stimulation on symptomatic behavior
has been variously assessed. There are references to a decline in the
frequency of stuttering associated with excitement, fear, anger, raised
voice, various drugs, or frequently as the result of the use of *mild* narcotics
or a small amount of alcohol (Bloodstein, 1949; Arnold, 1970b). However,
Hennig (1959) concludes from data on stuttering children that every excitement exacerbates stuttering regardless of whether it is caused by joy,
disappointment, or other factors.

PREVALENCE AND EXTENT OF STUTTERING

Even if meticulous and comprehensive research concerned with the
prevalence and extent of stuttering is lacking up to the present time, it is
agreed that stuttering is a disturbance of speech that occurs in people in
all the lands of the world (Sheehan, 1970b). Accordingly, a number of
questions are raised. What is the incidence of stuttering in a particular
country? At what age do symptoms of stuttering first appear? Or, how
many people subsequent to a short period of stuttering overcame it and,
above all, by what means? And in all of this there is the difficult question
of how satisfactory the answers are. This is not explained by the problem
of definition, which was mentioned previously. Rather, in the investigations of different authors there is considerable variation in the criteria for
self-differential diagnosis as between normal and abnormal speech disfluencies. Thus, comparison of the data is difficult. Van Riper (1971) makes
several additional critical points. There are not a few persons who on
interview will admit that they have a defect of speech but even if it is
stuttering do not want to be labeled "stutterer." Another problem in
epidemiological research is the inconsistency with which symptoms manifest themselves. This is especially so at an early age when there are
intermittent completely symptom-free periods that are not just exceptions
to the rule. For this reason many stutterers go unrecorded because their
symptoms appear only spasmodically (p. 37).

Nevertheless, two general kinds of statements are warranted:

- Stuttering commences in children more frequently than in adults.
  Based on documented research, Van Riper (1971) estimates the fre-

quency of stutterers in the general population to be 4%. The greatest percentages are to be found in the preschool years. The proportion of adult stutterers is less than 1%.

- Most stuttering is conspicuous after early childhood. Stuttering symptoms first appear before the age of 8 in 70 to 90% of stutterers.

As these overall data concerning age distribution show, the number of *spontaneous remissions* is considerable, even if these data derive from extraordinary variations in investigations (Sheehan & Martyn, 1966, 1967). There is obviously only a small number of stutterers who retain their symptoms throughout life. Yet spontaneous improvement appears to be dependent on several characteristics of the symptom picture (Martyn & Sheehan, 1968). Thus, the kind of speech difficulties at the onset of the disorder is significant. Clear repetition of syllables (clonic symptom picture) is more prognostic than blockages (tonic stuttering). The milder the disturbance the greater is the probability that it will subside without treatment. A lesser chance of spontaneous remission can be held out for those stutterers who are conscious of the disorder "stuttering" and have incorporated such a judgment into their self-concept. In contrast, a more favorable prognosis is likely for those who have not resigned themselves to their disorder and who concentrate on activities outside themselves.

Improvements in speech or complete correction have been shown to occur significantly in the periods from 11 to 14 and 19 to 22 years of age. This is a time of transition to a new stage of life. If the stuttering persists beyond age 22, then the probability of spontaneous remission decreases with advancing age.

SUMMARY

We have dealt with the initial identification of stuttering. This generally occurs on the level of description of symptoms. Thus, clonic and tonic stuttering as well as combinations of both manifestations are differentiated. We have further endeavored to organize the various phenomena associated with stuttering by pointing out important and typical relations among idiosyncrasies of stutterers. Accompanying symptoms and typical speech characteristics as well as distinction of stuttering from other speech disorders were discussed. Consistency and the dependence of stuttering on regularly observable situations and on particular characteristics of the speech disorder were described. Certain entries are italicized in order to designate standard terms that will be useful in discussing development of concepts. In view of the wide variety of accepted clinical phenomena, this seemed to be definitely practical and necessary for understanding the subsequent chapters of this book. An analysis of the data concerned with prevalence and extent of stuttering, including special attention to the question of spontaneous remission, concludes the first chapter.

Chapter 2

Origin of Stuttering: Genetic and Somatic Hypotheses

INTRODUCTION

We shall begin this chapter with a descriptive exposition of the genesis and the development of stuttering in early childhood. The large number of scientific studies concerning the origin of stuttering makes a comprehensive review impractical. Any attempt to analyze current scientifically based positions is complicated by the number and contradictions of the hypotheses having to do with the causes of speech disorders. Questions about hereditary and organic origins have led to numerous empirical studies concerned with differentiating between the genetic and somatic evolution of stuttering. In the course of this chapter it will become clear that the search for causal conditions is not entirely confined to somato-genetic factors. There are increasing references to psychological factors determined by social environment. Nevertheless, this chapter will contain many assumptions that are very plausible in clarifying the origin of stuttering, especially those that deal with stuttering as a consequence of disordered perception. They will be treated in some detail.

THE ONSET OF STUTTERING

There is widespread opinion that the first indication of childhood stuttering is excessive speech repetitions, mostly with syllables (Van Riper, 1971) but also involving a mixture of whole words and syllables (Froeschels, 1952). The genesis of stuttering is largely characterized by clonic or cloniclike irregularities. In a report of 700 documented cases Froeschels (1948) noted only one case of unequivocal tonic blocking at the onset of stuttering.

In most cases the development of symptoms of conspicuous stuttering takes place rather imperceptibly to begin with. Froeschels supposes that approximately 80% of children between the ages of 2 and 4 go through a phase of conspicuously rapid speech. When speech irregularities appear along with this it is called *developmental stuttering*. Generally, there is a great deal of word and syllable repetition. According to Froeschels' investigations about 1.8% of the children retain conspicuous stuttering symptoms from this phase of developmental stuttering (1948). Froeschels also terms this developmental stuttering "physiological stuttering," although this nomenclature is not at all precise. We can observe speech disfluencies at any time of life (Böhme, 1977).

Normally, developmental stuttering fades away spontaneously after several months without the child having been called a conspicuous "stutterer." Dickson (1969) reports a ratio of nine spontaneous remissions to each case of continuing symptoms; Quarrington (1956) estimates spontaneous remission in 80% of cases of developmental stuttering.

Statistics indicate that most stutterers become conspicuously so for the first time between 3 and 5 years of age (Sheehan, 1970b). Seeman (1969) indicates that in his retrospective study of beginning stuttering the onset occurred between 3 and 6 years of age in 66% of the cases. Research is often undertaken to pinpoint the precise time when stuttering begins (Berry, 1938; Johnson, 1959; Morley, 1957; McDearmont, 1968), but such studies are hardly practical since we must generally depend on questionable interview data, asking questions of persons in charge of the child's upbringing or education who are already more or less distant in time from the "status nascend" of the disordered speech.

It has rarely been reported that stuttering commences immediately with the utterance of the first word by the child. Aron (1962) reports several exceptions. Johnson (1956c) stated that a minimum of 6 months elapses between the utterance of the first word and the first noticeable stuttering; in one case stuttering was noted at 10 months and in two other cases at least 4 months before the utterance of sentences. In all other cases studied by Johnson stuttering first appeared after the speaking of sentences (the median was 13 months before the first attempt to speak in a sentence).

Rarely are cases reported in which there is sudden onset of stuttering. Still, it does happen in connection with a "traumatic experience," such as bodily injury, maltreatment, sudden fright, sudden fall, the bite of an animal, etc. However, that stuttering is unequivocally attributable to such a cause cannot now be verified. It is very rarely observed that stuttering clearly begins in adulthood. Here, for the most part, stutterers or referring individuals indicate war or accident traumas, brain injuries, and fever illnesses as causal external factors (Peachers & Harris, 1946; Wallen, 1961).

THE COURSE OF EARLY CHILDHOOD STUTTERING

Time and time again researchers describe the course of the speech disorder as a sequence of successive stages. However, they differ considerably from one another, as the three examples briefly summarized here illustrate.

The best-known classification by stage of the development of stuttering is that of Bluemel (1935), who distinguished between primary and secondary stuttering. Early childhood stuttering was labeled primary and a markedly pronounced symptom picture was classified as secondary.

Froeschels (1964) described seven developmental stages of stuttering: syllable and word repetition in normal speech tempo without tension (largely a clonic symptom type in stage 1); syllable and word repetition in normal speech tempo without tension and with increased tonic symptoms in a context of predominantly clonic ones (stage 2); syllable and word repetition in normal speech tempo with mild tension, clonic and clonic-tonic symptom type (stage 3); syllable and word repetition with tension and moderately increased speech tempo, clonic and clonic-tonic symptom type (stage 4); increasing acceleration of speech and increased tension in speaking, clonic or clonic-tonic symptom type (stage 5); increasing tension accompanying syllable and word repetition and now including significant slowing down of speech tempo and with it increasing tonic-clonic symptoms (stage 6); symptom picture marked by prolongation of sounds, severe tension, difficulties in articulation, as well as irregular breathing, decelerated speech, and increased tonic symptoms along with clonic and clonic-tonic types (stage 7).

The four-stage sequence described by Bloodstein (1960b) is our third example. Stage 1 is marked by periodic stuttering. The child stutters in situations of great stress, a consequence of agitation. Syllable and word repetitions occur primarily at the beginning of sentences and the child is not aware of speech deviations. In stage 2 an awareness of the disorder appears while the stuttering becomes chronic, which gives rise to severe emotional strain. The child stutters on nouns, verbs, and adjectives within sentences, increasing in stressful situations and with more rapid speech. In stage 3 situation dependency, situation variability, and consistency effects are observed; word paraphrasing and substitution first appear. Finally, in stage 4 conspicuous behaviors emerge such as the avoidance of speech and speech situations. Speech and situational anxieties appear; stuttering is expected and avoided. Word substitutions and paraphrasing are resorted to with increasing frequency; this is the stage of marked stuttering.

These authors refer to the didactic function of these or similar stage sequences. Furthermore, they believe that such an approach assists in choosing therapies suited to the particular stage. But others disagree. Widlak (1977) considers the stage concept to be of little value either in designating a particular stage in the course of a client's stuttering or in its application to therapy. The conditions related to the development of the disorder are so complex, each case having its own individual characteristics, that more often than not the specification of a stage is invalid. Widlak believes that the assignment of a stage to a client is risky, inasmuch as such "labeling" impedes meticulous observation and leads to overlooked signs (p. 31).

Van Riper (1971) especially criticizes the single-dimensional approach of most descriptions of the course of stuttering. He acknowledges that at one time he mistakenly supported the notion of a *single* typical course (1963). Based on his own long-time studies he now believes that four typical courses (tracks) of development can be extrapolated from his data.

In his description of courses of development Van Riper (1971, pp. 103–107) distinguishes between originating and developmental characteristics:

Developmental track I
Onset: Between two and one-half and four years of age; gradual and cyclic spontaneous remission; syllable repetition; no tension or tremor in talking; stuttering on important and initiating words predominates. Normal speech is present; no expectancy of stuttering; no feeling of inferiority about speech; no anxiety; there is a willingness to speak.

Course: Syllable repetition increases in frequency and rapidity; syllable repetition leads to prolongation of sounds; prolongation of syllables associated with tension and with quaking of the voice; conscious "struggle" against stuttering; frustrations set in; great increase in tension; contortions of the face; retrials of producing speech after stuttering; increasing fear before a speaking situation, before uttering words and sounds, poor eye contact; the stuttering child tries to conceal his speech difficulties; the typical repetitious and prolongation characteristics of stuttering and occasional hurried speech is the core behavior (predominant clonic and clonic-tonic symptom pattern).

Developmental track II
Onset: Utterance of whole sentences although they are not very fluent; stuttering is continuous without any periods of spontaneous remission; poor articulation, speech revisions, syllable

and word repetitions and gaps appear; for the time being, no tensions or tremors. Stuttering occurs on first words and long words; interruptions by gaps within sentences, no disfluency; no awareness, no frustration, no feeling of inferiority, no fear; willingness to talk.

Course: First of all rapidity of speech increases as does the frequency of deviations; a beginning awareness of the disorder and a feeling of inferiority as a consequence of frustrating attempts to control stuttering; increase of frequency of nonfluencies; more syllabic repetitions, also more syllables in a word; occasional fears of situations, though not of words and sounds; increased rapidity of repetition of long strings of syllables and accompanying jerkiness; good eye contact; no change in attempts to conceal; output of speech increases (clonic symptom picture with less prolongation of sounds but also tonic features).

Developmental track III

Onset: After period of beginning fluent speech sudden onset often after a drastic (traumatic) event; steady development of speech with few short periods of remission; normal articulation; child is intent upon slow careful rate; unvoiced prolongations before blocks accompanied by tension and tremor; longer periods of normal speech; from the beginning, awareness of difficulty, fear of words and situations.

Development: At first insignificant change in symptoms, small increase in frequency of errors; word retrials increase; longer lip protrusions and tongue fixations appear; unvoiced prolongations especially with initial sounds; increased tremor involving all imitation; tension of the mandible; marked frustration; prominence of interruptor devices; rate slows; more hesitancy and refusal to talk; intense fear of particular words and sounds needed for conversation; a variety of aids to talking (starters, expletives, paraphrasing); bizarre tension patterns; output of speech decreases, poor eye contact, normal speech is hesitant; frequent nonvocalized blockings (predominantly tonic features).

Developmental track IV

Onset: Late, usually after age 4; sudden appearance of disorders and continuous with spontaneous remissions. Normal articulation and rate; stutters mainly at beginning of words, many repetitions. Periods of fluent speech; nevertheless, conspicuous accompanying symptoms appear such as secretion of saliva, insertion of grunting sounds, exaggerated lip and tongue actions, grinding of teeth, marked activity of facial muscles during pauses in talking; highly aware although no frustration, little fear and willing to talk.

Development: The number of instances increases; little change in frequency but symptoms become more conspicuous; frequency increases with attempts to achieve fluency; slight tendency to avoid talking situations; participates in conversation; good eye contact, very aware of stuttering, little variability or change in stuttering behavior (tonic or clonic).

Van Riper arrived at these four tracks after long-time monitoring of 44 stutterers. Nevertheless, he admits it is likely that there will be additional individual courses of development. He himself has been able to assign only two-thirds of 300 clients to one of these four tracks (more or less unequivocally) (1971).

SEX-SPECIFIC DISTRIBUTION OF STUTTERING

The number of male stutterers exceeds females very significantly. Although, here too, the higher incidence rates vary from study to study, the conclusion of unequal relation between the sexes holds. Most investigations indicate the greater number of male stutterers to be in a ratio of about 3 (or 4) to 1 (e.g., Nadoleczny, 1926; Yates, 1970; Andrews & Harris, 1964).

We still lack a definitive explanation for this sex-specific distribution. Nevertheless, there is a formidable array of tentative hypotheses to explain the phenomenon. Thus, Goldman (1965, 1967) conjectures that the genesis of stuttering in little boys is fostered by the greater demands on them for achievement and by their stricter rearing. Tunner (1974) questions this. He, too, found more stuttering boys than girls but among the kibbutz children studied in Israel, where rearing practices for both sexes are almost identical. A promising explanatory possibility is suggested by the observation that girls acquire earlier and better speech facility and knowledge than boys (Van Riper, 1971).

Indications of the validity of the assumption that sex-associated differences may influence the origin of stuttering follow from the experiments of Bachrach (1964) and Stassi (1962). The former showed that delayed auditory feedback (DAF) elicited more disfluencies in male student subjects than females. (In DAF speech is fed back over earphones with a short time delay. Under the influence of the delayed feedback, the talker's speech is greatly distorted. There are interruptions and blockages in fluency that are similar to stuttering. We shall return to DAF later in the chapter.) Stassi found that under experimentally induced conditions of stress males had more blockages than females. At present, Van Riper holds that the best explanation of this difference lies in the assumption that there is a dispositional, possibly genetically determined, and a constitutional factor characterized by less stable neuromuscular development of the speech control system of males. Unfortunately, there is no empirical evidence for such an interpretation.

FAMILIAL OCCURRENCE OF STUTTERING

A large number of publications deal with the heredity of stuttering and possible congenitally determined predisposing conditions. Such investigations were once concerned with families in which at a given time and/or in the course of several generations specific behavioral signs or organic findings were present. For example, Wepman (1939) found that in 68% of families in which there was a stutterer there were other persons who had more or less fixed stuttering symptoms. For 51% of his stuttering clients Bryngelson (1935) found there were stuttering relatives. In a very careful study Andrews and Harris (1964) presented additional data. Their findings indicate the following probabilities that a family member of a stutterer will also stutter: mother, 5%; father, 19.1%; female and male siblings, 8.4 and 20%, respectively. Here, too, note the preponderance of male stutterers. All told, these authors found stuttering relatives in 38% of families in which there was a stutterer, as against 1.4% where there was no stutterer in the family. Although these and similar data of other authors seem to argue for a genetic basis for stuttering, most authors are rather hesitant to make such an assertion. In general it is debatable whether familial stuttering, as is the case in other behaviors, is not also a product of the learning process transmitted over generations (see Beech & Fransella, 1971, for a discussion of imitative learning).

This line of argumentation needs to be somewhat qualified by research on twins, which generally seeks to assess the influences of heredity and environment on the development of behavioral characteristics. In research on twins, data usually are gathered and compared concerning groups of identical and fraternal twins who have been reared in the same environment as well as groups of identical twins who have been reared together and separately (Lenz, 1970). Until now the interesting finding of many investigations has been that stuttering symptoms are observed much more often in twins than in other children at the same age. Furthermore, it has been found that there are more stutterers among identical than fraternal twins. Nelson, Hunter, and Walter (1945) found that among 200 twin pairs (131 fraternal and 69 identical) stutterers appeared in 22.7% of the identical and 14.8% of the fraternal twins. With almost no exception both of the identical twins stuttered, while in almost all cases of the fraternal twins only one stuttered. Luchsinger (1959) reported similar observations. Graf (1956), on the other hand, could not confirm these findings. In his study of 552 twin pairs he found 21 individual stutterers; only one of the identical pairs and two of the fraternal pairs exhibited actual coincidental speech disorders. But the possible coincidental presence of the disorder in identical twins does not quite support an unconditional hypothesis of a genetically determined predisposition to stuttering. There is much evidence that because of the marked common characteristics of identical twins we can expect more similar environmental shaping and rearing methods than with fraternal twins.

At present, statements neither about dominance or recessivity nor about possible polygenetic transmission of stuttering are warranted. Investigations of separately reared identical twins are lacking. As of now heredity of stuttering is neither unequivocally documented nor precluded.

ORGANIC CAUSES

Time and again organic factors are reported to play a preponderant role in the origin and development of stuttering. Most of these assumptions are hardly ever validated. They must therefore be considered speculative and not very substantive. Nevertheless, assessment of somatic factors is absolutely essential in the framework of differential diagnosis since in an individual case the cause of stuttering may be definitely organic. Speech disturbances are seen especially in cases of injuries to the brain and skull. Also, early childhood brain injuries (for example, following premature or forceps delivery) are found more frequently in stutterers than in normal-speaking persons (Böhme & Botzer, 1975; Böhme, 1966). Stuttering can also occur along with cerebral motor disturbances, as in, for example, hemiplegia, athetosis, and chorea (Böhme, 1966). And, finally, injurious accidents and brain damage can give rise to stuttering.

Stuttering and the Electroencephalogram

There have been a number of investigations dealing with the differences between stutterers and nonstutterers in electrical activity of the brain, in which the assumption is advanced that stuttering can be traced to an organic disturbance in the brain. However, the results relative to frequency vary considerably. Moreover, about 15% of all "normal" individuals show "abnormal" electroencephalograms (EEGs), especially if they are stimulated by flashes of light or are under induced hyperventilation (Van Riper, 1971). Among stutterers Landolt and Luchsinger (1954) found extensive, inconspicuous EEGs, while among clutterers (see Chapter 1) they found significant deviations in 90% of the cases. Gumpertz (1961) reported "pathological findings" in about 35% of his cases (stutterers and clutterers). In a large-scale investigation by Schönhärl and Bente (1960) of 400 admissions 54% exhibited a stuttering dysrhythmia and of these 32% showed unequivocal "pathologic" findings. Schmoigl and Ladisich (1967) tried to distinguish before examination between clutterers and stutterers with identifiable cerebral damage. The results showed that of the "pure" stutterers 10% had inconspicuous EEGs and 52% had "pathologic" ones.

This suggestion of apparent unequivocal results must, however, be interpreted with caution. Especially pertinent is the report of experiments by Andrews and Harris (1964). EEG curves of 30 pairs of children (normal-speaking versus stuttering) were judged by experts who did not know to which children (stuttering or nonstuttering) the curves applied. They found no differences. Neither were any found when pairs of curves were selected randomly and the experts were asked to indicate which belonged to stutterers or nonstutterers. These findings suggest that the scientific basis of EEG-based classification is open to question. That there is a preponderance of abnormal EEG findings among stutterers must be viewed with extreme reservation in any case.

This also goes for continually revived speculation concerning the correlation between epilepsy and stuttering, often based only on isolated observations. Several cases are described where stuttering was observed following epilepsy (Gens, 1951, and others). However, a direct relation, even when it exists, is generally confined to isolated cases. Also West's speculation (1958) that "pyknolepsie" (a mild form of petit-mal epilepsy) is causally related to stuttering has been repeatedly questioned. Hamre and Wingate (1967) have shown that there is substantial lack of relation between "petit-mal" and stuttering.

Cerebral Dominance and Speech Competence

As early as 1911 Stier pointed out that speech disorders such as stuttering were probably due to a unilateral defect of cerebral dominance. Normally, the left hemisphere is dominant and synchronizes motor impulses of both hemispheres, enabling integrated linguistic, auditory, or visual activity. The crossover in the medulla oblongata of the bulk of the nerve fibers of the motor system results in left-side dominance for right-handedness and (rarely) right-side dominance for left-handedness. If dominance of one or the other hemispheres is disturbed and ambivalence results, then disturbance of coordination follows. This also affects speech capability. Normally, the motor speech center, the center that controls motor speech activity, is located in the left half of the brain in the lower frontal convolution (Broca's area). A lesion in this area results in a speech disturbance (so-called *motor aphasia*), although individual musculature involved in speech is still innervated, and chewing, swallowing, whistling, and singing are possible. What is exclusively lacking for the production of speech is the necessary systematic coordination of the muscles involved in speech. As a rule left-handed persons (about 5% of the population) develop such a speech disturbance with a lesion in the right hemisphere, in contrast with right-handed persons who do so with a lesion in the left hemisphere. During the past few decades these findings having to do with handedness and ambidexterity and their possible relation to speech disturbances have stimulated a great number of investigations (Travis, 1931, 1951; Beech & Fransella, 1971).

From the evidence at hand it has been suggested that stutterers more frequently than nonstutterers are either left-handed or have been coerced into right-handedness while growing up. Bryngelson and Rutherford (1937) have shown that stutterers are ambidextrous four times more frequently and have been changed to right-handedness eight times more frequently than nonstutterers. However, Van Dusen (1939) and Daniels (1940) could find no significant relation between left-handedness and stuttering. Andrews and Harris (1964), too, found no difference in hand dominance between stutterers and nonstutterers. There is still a great deal of contradictory evidence concerning this problem (Johnson, Darley, & Spriestersbach, 1963).

Only recently has the theory of cerebral dominance and its significance for the etiology of stuttering acquired a new impetus. The methodology for determination of hemispheric dominance has been refined. For example, Wada and Rasmussen (1960) have developed a test that makes possible a determination from coordinated cortical impulses of the part played in speech and hand skills of left and right centers (so-called Wada Test). Subjects are given an injection of sodium amytol into the carotid artery. During this procedure involvement of arteries leading to the dominant hemisphere resulted in a transient paralysis of speech capability much like a motor aphasia in its symptoms. In addition, there was a disturbance of hand coordination on the contralateral side. Conversely, when blood was routed to the nondominant side aphasia and discoordination did not occur.

Jones, a neurosurgeon, administered the Wada Test to four adult stutterers with fixed symptoms (1966, 1967). To his surprise he found after injection of one or the other arteries that all four patients showed a transient aphasia as well. He concluded from this that stutterers have bilateral control of speech and this apparently results in interference phenomena. After operating on one of the hemispheres for brain pathology Jones found all four were symptom free. A subsequent administration of the Wada Test revealed that all four patients showed aphasia-like symptoms with injection of sodium amytol in the artery that supplied the nonoperated hemisphere.

A number of other investigations in recent decades involving the Wada Test as well as brain surgery lend substantial support to Jones' hypotheses (summarized by Van Riper, 1971; also by Lebrun and Bayle, 1973). With regard to ambilateral central dominance, Branch, Milner, and Rasmussen (1964) using Wada techniques showed that a large number of clients had either left or bilateral representation of speech. If there is clear difficulty in responsiveness (hence dominance) of the motor centers, then serious consequences in motor as well as linguistic capability result. These ideas were further documented in the report of the Brussels Symposium (Lebrun & Hoops, 1973).

The use of the Wada Test is not without risk. In about 3% of the persons on whom the test was used the examination ended in death (Van Riper, 1971). This fact alone is sufficient ground for abandoning the test, especially since risk-free methods for determination of hemisphere dominance are available.

Another test for determination of cerebral dominance is the Phi Test. The phi phenomenon occurs when points of light are presented successively with increasing rapidity so that an impression of movement results (Wertheimer, 1925). Jasper (1932) suggested that the direction in which the movement is perceived is at the same time an indication of the dominant hemisphere; right-handers (left-dominant) perceive movement to the right, left-handers (right-dominant) see movement to the left of the alternating flashes of light. Ambidextrous individuals experience an inconstant perception sometimes to one side, then to the other. The latter observation has been supported by investigations of stutterers (Beech & Fransella 1971, p. 82). Nevertheless, further research is necessary since there has not been sufficient application of scientific criteria to the contexts in which these investigations have been carried out.

Another means for the ascertainment of hemisphere dominance has been the possible diagnosis of auditory debility in one or the other side. Several connections to stuttering have been observed. Rosenzweig (1951) believes that dominance of one of the cochleas can be established with demonstration of better auditory ability in the corresponding ear. Curry and Gregory (1969) found that stutterers more frequently than normal-speaking persons heard better with the left ear than the right; when this was not the case the difference in the quality of hearing between the left and the right was much less for stutterers than for normal talkers. The authors assume that this is evidence for ambilaterality. Further research suggests that these findings are significant. Tomatis (1954) stated that 90% of the stutterers he studied had a hearing loss in the ear that should have been their preferred ear. He later claimed that stutterers controlled their speech with the ear that did not lead to the dominant auditory center (1963). Thus, they had to transfer to the other hemisphere the feedback information that they received from their own speech. This resulted in prolonged transfer time similar to the delayed auditory feedback that, as we noted previously, causes considerable speech disturbances. Tomatis' hypothesis has not been supported by further research. Nevertheless, it is extremely important in the general framework of investigations pointing to the relation of feedback to stuttering. We shall turn to these in detail in the sections that follow.

Stuttering and Disturbed Perception

In order to coordinate the flow of speech efficiently the talker requires continuous information on how well he or she is doing with what he or she has said and is saying. This self-control of the act of speaking is possible over a considerable array of feedback circuits of the perceptual system. First, those gross feedback channels can be distinguished which conduct the signals of vocal output to the central integration and control centers: auditory feedback to the ears by bilateral air conduction, by bilateral bone conduction, and by bilateral connective tissue. Additional feedback speech signals come from the sensation of movement (kinesthetic feedback), from sensations of touch (tactile feedback), as well as from the sensations of the proprioceptive reflexes (from internal stimuli). Given these many feedback mechanisms, it is reasonable to assume that various disturbances can ensue. Hence, the process of integration is made difficult when feedback information arrives at the left or right hemisphere quite asynchronously or when interferences occur, which result in differing transmission times over the various nervous channels. It is obvious that as a consequence of such disorders integration of feedback signals is not possible and as a result discoordination of speech and with it stuttering ensues.

These hypotheses have gained increasing plausibility since speech disturbance can be evoked artificially in normal-speaking individuals by inducing disturbance of perception of their own speech. First, we shall describe more specifically the conditions and features of this "artificial" stuttering in normal talkers and then advance several hypotheses concerning the genesis of stuttering (stuttering as a perceptual defect).

The Lee Effect

If we present their own utterances to nonstuttering normally fluent talkers over earphones with a time delay of less than a tenth of a second they hear their own speech like an echo. Then considerable talker disfluency similar to that of a stutterer occurs. This phenomenon of experimentally produced speech disturbance has been named for its discoverer, B. S. Lee. In 1951 Lee reported on the disordering effect of delayed auditory feedback (DAF) on the fluency of the speech of normal talkers (see also Black, 1951). Even when the speech of normal talkers under conditions of DAF were found by spectrographic analysis to be convincingly similar to that of stutterers in a study by Rawnsley and Harris (1954) there was not up to that time any agreement as to whether the analogy about conditions and manifestations of both phenomena was real (Soderberg, 1968, 1969). Interesting comparisons are in order.

The speech disturbances manifested by normal talkers under conditions of delayed feedback are quite typical and although there are temporary individual differences they are easily elicited (Röck, 1977). Sound and syllable repetitions occur and blockages are observable. Vowels are prolonged significantly. Rapidity of speech is generally subject to marked fluctuations from very rapid to dragging. Usually, intensity of sounds, pitch, and effort, especially precise articulation, increase (so-called Lombard Effect; Lombard, 1910). These are presumably countercontrol reactions, attempts by the organism to overcome difficulty by drowning out with increased sound intensity the prolonged production of the fed back sounds, a thoroughly ineffective undertaking since the variations in sound intensity are likewise fed back over the earphones. The length of time delay required to produce maximum disturbance varies with the age of the subject. For young adults (to age 30) the delay time to produce the severest disturbance lies somewhere between .16 and .22 seconds. For older and younger persons a much longer delay time is required to produce the maximal effect: between the ages of 4 and 9 about .6 seconds, older people between 60 and 80, about .4 seconds (MacKay, 1968; Buxton, 1969).

There are considerable individual differences. There are older and very young people who experience maximum disturbance with relatively short time delays (Smith & Tierney, 1971). In general, though, it can be confidently asserted that speech disturbances evoked by DAF (rapidity, distortion of speech) are more severe and more evident the longer the time delay required to produce maximum disturbance. The critical value for females is longer. However, contrary to the evidence of DAF effects, males appear to be more prone to speech disturbances (Bachrach, 1964). We have already discussed the relation of stuttering to sex difference and have there looked into and commented upon the greater possibility of an unstable constitutional neuromuscular speech control system in males.

In research on delayed speech feedback varying emotional reactions are frequently observed. Some subjects manifest strong emotional excitement, which is also evident in measurements of skin resistance (Haywood, 1963). Others show minimal emotional changes. The extent of a subject's affective involvement is likely to depend on his or her capacity for tolerating a speech disturbance or for controlling it (for example, by training). Here too, precise data are lacking. Emotionally affected individuals seem to retain the induced speech disfluency many minutes more (some much longer) after the conclusion of the experiment. Tiffany and Hanley (1956) reported a case in which an obvious special fear of a particular word had developed. After the examination the subject avoided using the word. The Lee Effect frequently gives rise to marked disorder especially in children. With them the disturbances are much more widely exhibited than with older persons. This is probably due to the as yet undeveloped confidence of younger people in the motor speech act (Chase, Sutton, First, & Zubin, 1961).

The speech-disturbing effects of DAF are significantly less under conditions of simultaneous stimulation and activity, much as with stuttering (Chapter 1), as, for example, writing from a text (Smith, 1962; Smith & Smith, 1962). Also under DAF conditions when some means is inserted to accomplish transfer, that is, concentration on the part of a normal talker away from auditory attention to the signal-delayed feedback and to other stimuli, fluent speech results (Röck, 1977). Similar effects are produced by jamming the DAF signal or by complicating perceptibility, for example, by simultaneous insertion of white noise. White noise is a mixture of noise produced by a tone generator in which the acoustic energy is distributed equally over the entire frequency spectrum. In this and experiments similar to DAF it is presented to subjects over earphones. (Compare to "masking," Chapter 6.) Generally, the explanation of these effects is that the talker is more or less diverted from auditory self-control of his or her speech and is thus forced to control vocal output over internal proprioceptive and tactile channels. Consequently, the ensuing auditory interference is less significant. "All steps and factors that in any way increase the attentiveness and latitude for speech behavior in the DAF situation result in a diminution of the effect to the extent that transfer to proprioceptive-tactile control of speech can be accomplished" (Röck, 1977, p. 70).

Stuttering and Interference by Auditory Feedback

As we have already pointed out, the effect on normal speech of delayed feedback is similar in symptoms to those of stuttering. This has stimulated the formulation of hypotheses that view the origin and maintenance of stuttering as a disturbance of the self-control mechanisms of speech produced by a defect in the perceptual system. Among the first advocates of this point of view were Cherry and Sayers (1956; also Cherry, Sayers, & Marland, 1956), who investigated such a hypothesis by interrupting the perceptual loop. They asked their clients to repeat as quickly as possible the words of a text invisible to them read by a therapist (so-called "shadow speech," see Chapter 6). The authors believed that this procedure diverted the attention of the stutterer from his or her own speech and thereby eliminated the assumed disturbing influence of the feedback of speech transmitted by air and bone conduction. In so doing they were able to reduce stuttering considerably and in some cases to eliminate it completely.

Cherry and Sayers were also able to reduce stuttering symptoms by presenting a loud noise while the stutterer was talking and/or requesting him or her to talk in only a whisper, seeking thereby to eliminate perception of loud speech sounds. The results of this investigation were considered to support the claim that stuttering is a defect of the perception of self-produced low-frequency sounds. In another experiment, in order to determine the relative contribution of air and bone conduction to the speech disturbance, Cherry and Sayers interrupted auditory feedback by air conduction by securely blocking both ears. The stuttering persisted at its former level of severity, which the authors claimed to be evidence that the bone conduction channel was the one involved in the interference (see, however, Macioszek, 1973). The authors then masked out the acoustic speech coupling of stutterers with white noise. This masking resulted in substantial improvement of the speech behavior of the stutterers. The reduction in the number of repetitions was increased with increasing intensity of the white noise. Often complete disappearance of the disorder was observed. These findings were confirmed by subsequent research (Stromsta, 1958; Maraist & Hutton, 1957). Cherry and Sayers presented this as evidence for their previously formulated assumptions.

Van Riper (1971) supplemented and refined these ideas. It is his opinion that speech production of a child during the period of speech acquisition is predominantly controlled by hearing. In the course of further speech development these control functions are taken over by superficial (touch and contact sensations) and deeper senses (positional and kinesthetic) concerned with the speech mechanism. The auditory channels are increasingly reserved for reception of external stimuli, for "intellectual" control by the organism. This transfer of the control of speech output by superficial and deep senses (proprioceptive and tactile feedback) is gradually accomplished as the auditory feedback channel is used less and less for correction of errors (for example, in the learning of sounds). Discontinuance of auditory control takes place slowly and stepwise as the confidence of the child in his or her speech and articulation increases. In the transition, competition among the various feedback loops can increase the probability of disturbance, especially when incipient control of the speech mechanism by proprioceptive-tactile means occurs simultaneously along with auditory control by air and bone conduction. Van Riper states that this accounts for the observation of developmental stuttering in almost 80% of all children. If auditory control of speech persists, speech disturbance (stuttering) ensues uninterruptedly. But, as a rule, there is spontaneous remission if perceptual control of proper speech by proprioceptive-tactile sensitivity is established. Adults ultimately control their speech almost exclusively by the superficial and deep sensations associated with the speech mechanism. Van Riper advances this view as a result of his observations of symptom-free speech of stutterers with masking by white noise and the observed absence of stuttering in deaf persons as typical examples.

The significance of proprioceptive and tactile sensory involvement in symptom-free speech is also supported by research in which the feedback channel is blocked as, for example, by anesthesia (McCroskey, 1958; Ringel & Steer, 1963; Schliesser & Coleman, 1968).

The Effects of Delayed Speech Feedback on Stuttering

When stutterers are asked to talk under conditions of delayed auditory feedback they are relieved of symptoms (Nessel, 1958; Lotzmann, 1961). Typical abnormal breathing and associated movements also diminish. This effect can be interpreted as being due to the difficulty of self-control of speech caused by the DAF signal and the necessity for the stutterer to shift his or her concentration to kinesthetic control. Similarly, typical speech abnormalities occur to a nonstutterer under DAF conditions (Macioszek, 1973; so-called "negative" Lee Effect; Lotzmann, 1961). The considerable improvement in speech behavior of stutterers noted with DAF is dependent on intensity of sounds (masking conditions) as well as the length of time delay (diverting conditions). Macioszek (1973) has shown that only in cases of moderate stuttering is maximal symptom reduction achieved by greater sound intensity—due to masking of auditory feedback to the ear and bone conduction. With severe stutterers moderate sound intensity results in maximum symptom-free speech output and loud sounds result in no improvement. The claim of Cherry and Sayers that bone conduction is the distinctive channel involved in the disturbance is not supported by Macioszek.

Additional Findings

Information about the neural structure and function of the speech mechanism is sparse. However, in the last few decades research in simulation of these processes through cybernetic modeling has led to substantial advances (Fairbanks, 1954; Mysak, 1960; Früh, 1965; Röck, 1977). Until now, this promising work has been admittedly speculative as to whether or just where there is possible relevance to the feedback interferences that have been described. Research using DAF and white noise suggests that the feedback interferences are not a defect of only one feedback channel but are the interfering information of various channels and the resulting difficulty of processing and dealing with it effectively (Widlak, 1977). A description of several illustrative investigations on this point follows.

Sutton and Chase (1961) and Webster and Dorman (1970) found that insertion of white noise during intervals of silence of stutterers reduced speech disturbances as much as continuous noise. For an explanation of this phenomenon these investigators drew on the work of Djupesland (1964, 1965) as well as that of Shearer and Simmons (1965) having to do with the action of the middle-ear muscles. The contraction of these muscles preceded vocalization by 65 to 100 milliseconds and was also observed in subjects who were expecting a sudden noise. These contractions obviously protect the sense organ from overload by an impulse stimulus (also by the speaker's voice). Webster and Lubker (1968) claimed that contraction of these muscles occurs along with the insertion of white noise during silent intervals in speech, which at the onset of speech checks the potential interference from auditory feedback by the impending action of the contraction. If white noise is inserted in silent intervals, contraction (as protection from overload) occurs. It is being increasingly suggested that with such auditory feedback, conditioning of the onset of speech takes place and is generalized to the speech itself. This seems to explain the therapeutic effects of masking on stuttering (see Chapter 6). "Training" the middle-ear muscles elevates the threshold of perception of auditory stimulation by one's own speech.

It may be that in normal speech development with the increasing significance of external acoustic stimuli the threshold of perception for the acoustic signals of one's own speech is elevated (spontaneous remission in developmental stuttering). It may also be that the threshold for the perception of stutterers' own speech remains depressed when they constantly try to talk normally. If the threshold remains depressed the competition among various auditory and other feedback channels becomes crucial and appropriate integration is made more difficult.

Additional experimental findings on DAF with stutterers and normal talkers have been presented by Stromsta (1959, 1972) and Mahaffey and Stromsta (1965). Bekesy (1932) first demonstrated that simultaneous presentation of air- and bone-conducted signals can produce cancellation of the sensation of a tone. Then by appropriate methods it is possible to extinguish the movement of the basilar membrane (caused by the bone-conducted sound) by introducing similar or opposing air-conducted sounds. Stromsta was able to show that there was a significant difference between stutterers and nonstutterers with respect to this "interaural phase difference." Using special apparatus a tone of fixed frequency and amplitude was presented to an ear by bone conduction (by way of the incisors of the subject) and by air conduction. Manipulation of the phase angle of the tone could cancel its sensation. These differences between both ears obtained at the instant of elimination of the tonal sensation are considerably greater for stutterers than for nonstutterers. Reversing this effect the investigator could produce stuttering symptoms in nonstutterers by elevating the interaural phase difference. These findings further show clear and considerable differences in the speed of conduction over various feedback systems that are probably due to anatomical-physiological factors (constitutional differences). Since males show greater discrepancies in this regard it may also probably be an explanation for the unequal prevalence of stuttering between the sexes.

In summary, we can make the following points to suggest that a perceptual defect is a possible cause of stuttering:

• Almost all investigations show that reduction of speech disturbances of stutterers can be achieved by masking out the auditory feedback of the talker's own speech. This argues for a disturbing effect on speech if an auditory feedback circuit is unaffected. It has not been clearly determined to which of the feedback circuits this disturbing effect on integration of fed back signals can be attributed. Interaction of a complex nature probably needs to be considered. Stuttering persists with exclusive blocking of air conduction, which may be viewed as a sign of disordered bone conduction. The marked improvement in speech with whispering or with exposure to white noise points to the potential for disturbance resulting from the talker's own speaking of low-frequency sounds. Finally, varying delay times of DAF gives rise to individual maximum improvements, suggesting that causal factors related to temporal and neural competition among various feedback routes need to be considered.

- Speech disfluencies of normal talkers under various DAF conditions are significantly influenced as are stutterers by variations in the talking situation. We shall show later—and also in the following section— that specific features of the total social speaking situation need to be considered as explanations of the phenomenon of natural as well as "artificial" stuttering.

Comparison of DAF findings of speech disfluencies among normal talkers and with stutterers is difficult since hypotheses about long-time effects of DAF that occur in nonstutterers need to be examined. Also, the manner in which these feedback interferences affect coordination of muscle groups (disturbing ones) involved in the speech act has not yet been fully determined. In concluding we shall now consider several tentative hypotheses.

Stuttering as Neuromuscular Discoordination

That the causes, among others, of the tensions characteristic of stuttering are to be attributed to a possible desynchronization of cortical control impulses associated with muscle groups involved in the speech act has been suggested by several authors (Liebmann, 1903; Nadoleczney, 1926; Seeman, 1934, 1969; Brankel, 1959; Hartlieb, 1969; Fernau-Horn, 1969). According to Richter (1970), this can be reduced to five phenomena:

1. Speech impulses arrive too rapidly so that the musculature cannot keep pace.
2. Speech impulses are delayed, irregular, doubled, or as much as quadrupled for a time.
3. Phonation occurs with the desire to speak but the overexcited articulatory muscles are unable to react.
4. Articulatory musculature is activated, lips and tongue move but voice is lacking.
5. When activating conditions are extreme speech can be completely blocked so that impulses for phonation and articulation are blocked. Under subjective/objective pressure to speak the stutterer tries to force out the words with great muscular exertion—and really begins to stutter.

It is generally thought that in cases of somatic hyperactivity or instability the predisposition to muscle tension (especially of the breathing, larynx, and speech musculature) is increased. Schwartz (1977) sees a conditioned laryngospasm (reflexive laryngeal tension) as the main cause of stuttering. As a consequence of autonomic control in activating situations (especially with anxiety and stress) there is a sudden reflexive tensing of the vocal bands that is difficult to terminate. The stutterer cannot talk anymore because the vocal bands cannot be vibrated, as he or she would be able to do with regular expiration of air. The urge to expel the air only reinforces the tension of the vocal bands, which results in still more unsuccessful effort by the stutterer who wants to talk.

Psychological factors appear to be clearly involved in the hypotheses that stuttering is due to neuromuscular discoordination. If anxiety and stress are indeed causal factors leading, for example, to conditioned tension of the speech musculature (learned and stimulus dependent), then it is necessary to investigate more specifically the relation between environmental and somatic factors. The interdependence of socially induced anxiety and stress and the constitutional predisposition to tension have been studied, especially from the point of view of psychological theories. We shall discuss them in the next chapter in more detail.

SUMMARY

This chapter dealt with the origin and cause of stuttering. The characteristics of the disorder in its early stages of development were presented. That stuttering frequently occurs in families and that there are more male than female stutterers raises the question of the possibility that stuttering is inherited. This is not quite supported by the results of research in learning. In addition, explanations that emphasize various somatic factors are still not incontrovertible. Furthermore, EEG findings are not without criticism. A relation between cerebral dominance and speech competence is, to be sure, evident and generally accepted. The various theoretical deductions about cerebral dominance as a determinable cause for stuttering are not clearly and unequivocally established but are being examined.

Current hypotheses based on very careful research argue for the dependence on feedback processes of normal and disordered speech. Much has been made of the point that stuttering is associated with a desynchronization of feedback and coordinating processes. The plausibility of these assumptions is questioned, however, by findings of situation-dependent variability in stuttering such as significantly more fluent speech by stutterers of dialect, shadow speech, singing, and in talking to children and animals. Stuttering does not occur in these situations in which the talker's own speech definitely needs to be controlled over perceptual channels. This is weighty evidence that psychic variables are involved in the "organic defect" and for this reason it cannot be considered as the sole cause of stuttering (Tunner, 1974). This also clearly applies to hypotheses that argue for neuromuscular discoordination as a possible cause.

In the following chapter we shall attempt to cover hypotheses concerned with the significance of environmental factors involved in stuttering behavior. For this purpose we shall select among the many psychological explanatory views those that are based on widely accepted models and discuss their plausibility and their direct integration with the somatic-genetic hypotheses to which we have previously referred.

Development and Maintenance of Stuttering: Psychological Research and Interpretation

INTRODUCTION

In preceding chapters the prominent role of somatic factors in the origin of stuttering has been pointed out in some detail. And when we mentioned environmental factors it was not with the intent of viewing them as an explanation for the origin of stuttering. From the point of view of many medical opinions the question of interrelations between constitutional and environmental factors in the evolution of stuttering appears to have been unequivocally determined (hardly discussed and one-sided) to favor constitutional predisposition. Tunner (1974), however, considers such a one-sided determination "antiquated," the more so as current advances in research in the area of conditioning central and peripheral physiological processes allow insight into the diversity of possibilities for shaping and altering behavior precisely by mutual interdependence of somatic and specific environmental factors (also Birbaumer, 1975).

This chapter, accordingly, will consider the concepts and models that inquire chiefly into the validity of specific environmental factors involved in the origin and maintenance of stuttering. In this connection the focus is on theories that attempt to approach speech disorder with appeal to various learning paradigms as, for example, classical, operant, or instrumental conditioning and social learning by observation/imitation. The bases for various learning theories need not be repeated here; recommended to the reader are the following pertinent introductory works, for example: Foppa (1965), Angermeier (1972), Angermeier and Peters (1973), and Lefrancois (1976). For an understanding of the intepretations to follow we will briefly mention the basic formulations.

Various authors in introducing their attempts to present and to criticize psychological theories are in agreement about their description of the field; there are many different theories and they are constantly increasing. All told, the picture presented by these theories appears, at first glance, to be bewildering. This is not surprising. An agreed upon theoretical formulation is currently lacking. And although there are several basic agreements, the many controversial formulations have resisted integration.

We are thus restricted to a rather sketchy presentation of psychological interpretations. In so doing we shall elaborate aspects of various theories that point to integration and also examine propositions of particular authors when they are central to these ideas of integration. We think it essential that we consider orderly classifications that qualify as illustrative examples of theoretical points of view. What is more we shall evaluate their importance for the treatment of stuttering.

Because of their general significance precisely in regard to the criterion of relevance to therapy it is well to summarize the paradigms that grow out of the concepts of operant and classical conditioning. Of late, the significance of the reactions of the environment to stuttering has attracted increasing attention: this relates to so-called "diagnosogenic" theories supplemented in a narrow sense by concepts from learning theory. Here, and also in the context of our exposition, expansion of the basic concepts of powerful cognitive variables is involved. Generally speaking, the cluster of cognitive theories plays an important role in attempts at psychological interpretations. They shall be included here.

STUTTERING AS OPERANT BEHAVIOR

Attempts to explain stuttering based on learning theory frequently assume a disturbance of normal speech development, elucidated, for the most part, by typical consequences of reward and punishment. Such an attempt was undertaken by Shames and Sherrick (1963) and more recently by Shames and Egolf (1976). This operant explanation proceeds from the assumption that there is a continuous transition from normal speech to deviant speech and disfluencies diagnosed as "stuttering" (the so-called *continuity hypothesis*). Just as with fluent speech, stuttering is operantly determined. It is learned just as fluent speech is learned and its acquisition occurs essentially from conditions set by the social environment (reinforcement, punishment, modeling, instruction, etc.). Where stuttering is concerned there are no simple contingencies. Rather, complex and multiple patterns of reinforcement are responsible for the origin, development, and maintenance of stuttering.

Origin hypotheses: As children, we learn quite early to remain silent until our interlocutor has finished talking. We learn conversely that the silence of the other person is a signal for us to talk. Often, according to

Shames and Sherrick (1963), the talker intends *no* such signal. The silent interval is merely a pause for thinking. If we begin to speak during one of these pauses we are likely to be interrupted. If this happens often we integrate into our speech the sequence "onset of speech-pause ('Is the interlocutor speaking?') -speech ". We further learn that our own speech pauses (thought pauses) serve as similar signals for the interlocutor during which we insert word repetitions, word prolongations, and sounds such as "uh," "so," etc., as appropriate means for bridging the pause. These are all speech mannerisms that to a moderate degree characterize "normal" speech. The more extreme shaping of these disfluencies is the learning condition responsible for incipient stuttering by children.

Development hypotheses: The speech disfluencies that have been described are then tolerated largely by the persons responsible for rearing the child and, among other things, are judged to be the "natural difficulties" of a child learning to talk. It may be that this early acceptance of speech disturbance on particular occasions (such as sanction by parents when the child speaks at the same time) is a potentially positive reinforcer, which in the opinion of operant assumptions about learning can finally stabilize such disfluencies even if the sanctions are intermittent, that is, resulting in irregular consequences. As the child matures there are increasing social demands for improved speech. Since it is possible that the disfluencies are thoroughly fixed the efforts by the caretaker to modify the speech behavior are in many cases ineffective. The child is often punished or is threatened with punishment. Consequently, he or she makes use of accessory helpful devices such as finger snapping, tensing the face, nodding the head, foot stamping (so-called *associated movements*; Chapter 1). These trial-and-error expedients are rarely effective in overcoming stabilized speech disfluencies. But they are retained as part of stuttering symptomatology since their useful functions in improving speech are difficult to assess.

Maintenance of stuttering hypotheses: If the disturbance has become fixed a "secondary difficulty" can turn up. Such children are pitied, more attention is paid to them by the rearing person; they can use their stuttering to enforce their wishes. Stuttering leads to educational problems. The behavior is maintained while speaking situations are avoided. Consequently, these children miss many aversive experiences and cannot venture upon new learning. Thus, speech difficulties develop into a complex social behavior disorder that is under the control of firmly established intermittent active patterns of reinforcement. Although the hypotheses of Shames et al. have generated several therapeutic approaches (see Chapter 6), the evidence has yet to be produced that in the long run operant conditioning is responsible for the onset and maintenance of stuttering.

Nevertheless, in association with other concepts, this theory is significant, for example, in complementing the ideas that have to do with speech disfluencies and stuttering as consequences of arousal of emotional state.

EMOTIONAL AGITATION AND STUTTERING

Of the authors who conceive of stuttering as the result of processes of classical conditioning, Brutten and Shoemaker (1969) should be mentioned especially. They incline toward this view through their concept of the classical conditioning paradigm (Angermeier & Peters, 1973), to which they appeal in attributing the inability of a stutterer to speak fluently to conditioned negative emotions. To begin with the authors proceed from the normal speech habits and speech competencies of the child. Disfluencies in speech output that can be traced back to situations of stress and punishment occur sporadically. As a rule stress produces alterations in the autonomic system that can also result in blockages of speech. Such speech disturbances have been demonstrated experimentally with normal-speaking people using intermittent presentation of threatening stimuli and stressors (e.g., Siegel & Martin, 1968).

Brutten and Shoemaker believe that the sporadically occurring speech disfluencies are then fixed when the fear of stressful situations persists and in fact increase (with stutterers these situations may be signs from an interlocutor, expectation of failures in production of sounds, words, and parts of sentences, etc.). The state of emotional arousal aggravates poor coordination between breathing and speaking, leading to faulty thinking and finally to refusal to talk. All of these are typical fear reactions showing "involuntary reflexive qualities" (Tunner, 1974, p. 454), which lends credence to the hypothesis of constantly expanding classical conditioning. Every upcoming neutral stimulus that is associated with these original emotions can act as a conditioned stimulus for avoidance of talking.

Schwartz (1977) has currently contributed to further development of the thinking of Brutten and Shoemaker. In the previous chapter we commented briefly on his notion that stuttering is a consequence of a conditioned tensing of the larynx (laryngospasm). Schwartz claims that it is psychological stress that generates tension of the vocal bands and this triggers stuttering. He differentiates seven stress-producing stimuli that are responsible for laryngeal tension.

1. *Situational stress*: Some social stimuli are likely to demand symptom-free speech and to lead to intense anticipatory anxiety, giving rise to

stress reactions. Although these can vary among individuals, there are several situations that are typical for many stutterers (e.g., using the telephone, public speaking, speaking before a microphone or a camera).

2. *Word or sound stress*: There are particular syllables, parts of words, or words that the "experience" of the stutterer has tagged as especially "prone" to trigger stuttering. Almost all stutterers have specific word fears; they also try constantly to avoid these words. Some develop an amazing ability to substitute "easy" words for difficult ones in order to mask their stuttering. However, this is not always possible and stress reactions and stuttering take place.

3. *Authority-person stress*: Psychological stress often occurs when stutterers are talking to persons of higher social status. With people who are of equal or lesser status they speak markedly more fluently.

4. *Insecurity stress*: There are situations in which the stutterer feels insecure because he or she has had little or no experience of communication in them and feels incompetent to cope with them.

5. *Physiological stress*: If the general health of the stutterer is affected, for example, as a conseqence of illness or exhaustion, physiological stress can occur.

6. *Incident stress*: Stress can be triggered by an unexpected incident or traumatic event. Unnerving news and information can be the cause. (In such cases Schwartz also speaks of "Job's" stress.)

7. *Rapidity stress*: Stress can arise from talking too rapidly. According to Schwartz, this is the kind of stress in which the stutterer reverts to stuttering if he or she must persist in talking too slowly and deliberately.

Added to the predisposition for the onset of laryngeal tension related to one or more of these stress factors is the general "basic stress level" of stutterers. This is determined by the overall activating level (the extant muscle tension of the entire body). According to Schwartz, the vocal bands are acutely sensitive indicators of the basic stress level. With increased activation they are tightly tensed so that only a slight additional stress is required to trigger the conditioned tension when talking and thus bring on the stuttering.

In the course of development of their disorder stutterers seek ways by which they can gain control of negative emotions and consequently of speech disfluencies. They increasingly engage in kinds of behavior that allow them to avoid anxiety-producing stimuli and to withdraw from situations that are fraught with fear (escape behavior). These reactions can be verbal (e.g., altering choice of words) or nonverbal (e.g., finger snapping or fist clenching).

As these behavioral patterns become more prominent the onset and shaping of stuttering cannot be explained solely by classical conditioning but emerge through an operant learning process. This elaboration is termed a 2 Factor Theory (or a 2 process theory) of stuttering. It is derived mainly from the fundamental hypotheses of Mowrer (1956, supplemented, 1968). The attempt to explain the development of stuttering as rigorously behavioral based on a synthesis of stuttering phenomena from the point of view of both learning paradigms has retained its plausibility and several authors have subscribed to its integrative approach (Tunner & Florin, 1969; also Tunner, 1974). Nevertheless, the 2 Factor Theory is not without criticism. In fact, the developmental phenomena of stuttering (and the mechanism for its maintenance) can be described from the point of view of Brutten and Shoemaker as well as Mowrer. The answer to the question, as addressed by the operant concept, as to when and how stuttering begins is still purely hypothetical.

Van Riper (1971) cites several experimental findings countering the claim in the field that initial stuttering is a consequence of physiologic-motor activation by stress (the frequent typical result under experimental conditions of symptom reduction with easing of anxiety-producing and threatening stimuli; also Siegel, 1970; Goldiamond, 1965).

STUTTERING AS A CONSEQUENCE OF DIAGNOSIS

A committed opponent of the effort to explain stuttering on a purely medical-somatic basis is Johnson (1956b,c). He is equally vehement in opposing efforts to classify stuttering on the basis of neuroses, especially deep psychological concepts (also 1959). The very difficulties in determining the criteria for classifying symptoms of stuttering led him to the idea that the question of the differentiation of stuttering from nonstuttering, especially in the early stages of the development of stuttering, is central. From this Johnson, as did Shames (1968), states that in the development of a child's speech we cannot point convincingly to a significant difference between stuttering and nonstuttering children. He believes that assigning the deviant speech of a child to the category "stuttering" is in almost all cases done by laymen, mostly parents, and that they judge as "stuttering" disturbances that for the most part are like the speech nonfluencies of adults. Hence, the child's speech peculiarities are not the determining factor in a diagnosis of stuttering. Rather their evaluation is based on the naive criteria growing out of the experience with adults. For Johnson the problem of stuttering is that it gets diagnosed as such (the so-called *diagnosogenic theory*). Stuttering begins not before but first with and then after its diagnosis.

The diagnostic and with it the correctional reaction of the caretaker instills in the child the conviction that speech is difficult. Such children recognize that they are unable to speak properly but at the same time are aware that this behavior is demanded of them. From then there is intense awareness of the speech process. As difficulties are anticipated in talking special efforts to prevent them are resorted to and the groundwork is laid for their actual onset (anticipatory struggle reaction; Bloodstein, 1958; Wischner, 1952).

For Johnson (1956c, 1959) stuttering is avoidance behavior traceable to expectancy anxiety. The avoidance behavior caused by anticipatory fears is concerned, for example, with sounds, words, or various features of social speaking situations. Depending on his or her experiences (e.g., punishment, subjectively experienced distress with his or her own speech difficulties, feelings of tension and helplessness), the stutterer will be anxious to avoid the anticipated stuttering and this will be greater the greater the anxiety. Therefore stuttering will be equated with the attempts to avoid stuttering. Johnson describes the conditions for the maintenance of stuttering primarily in behavioral terms. Consistently and logically, as in the ideas described above, he stresses a social component, social diagnosis, in his explanatory model as a cause of speech disturbance. This has important consequences for therapeutic measures. Therefore, methods such as training for a realistic assessment of one's own speech competence, efforts to accept the disorder, and self-training under varying social circumstances are central to Johnson's concept of therapy.

Johnson's views illustrate the numerous variables that operate on the onset of stuttering. At the same time they constitute an important criticism by advocates of rigid learning theory. The question then is whether the formal language of functional behavior theory is sufficient to encompass the genuine context dependencies of the social behavior of stutterers, to adequately take into account norms and standards, as well as to specify behavioral objectives and expectations explicitly. Before we return to this question we shall next examine social aspects in somewhat less detail.

DIGRESSION: STUTTERING AS SOCIAL BEHAVIOR

In social groups the behavior of individuals is constantly judged according to norms and standards of the most discriminating kind. For membership in a particular social group a considerable number of specific rules of behavior are prescribed as appropriate to which an individual must accommodate his or her communication and ways of interacting. Above all, conversation serves as a means of reciprocal transmission of content between one who talks and one who listens. This communication can be described as a process in a system marked by numerous rules of behavior. The competence of an individual in communicating according to such rules is reflected in his or her immediate actual behavior. Contravention of these norms and rules results in rejection, termination of communication, loss of status, and isolation.

The stutterers constantly violate these conventional rules of communication. Their speech disorder marks them as substantially different from other people in an undesirable way. Therefore in social situations they struggle against isolation and loss of prestige, or they believe they must struggle against them. The basis for this is the fear of social rejection, the stigma of abnormality, and the anticipation of communicative incompetence (Perkins, 1965). Embarrassing and pained reactions of the listener generate intense fear reactions especially in those speaking situations in which punishment by the caretaker can be anticipated (Widlak, 1977). Then, typical customary behavior follows on the part of those who are conversing with the stutterer (Van Riper, 1971).

Caretakers for the most part are of the opinion that stutterers stutter because of "nervousness;" therefore, they need to be calmed. This opinion may also be traceable to their own experience that under stress fluent speech is difficult. Often it is helpful to suggest that the stutterer might relax and not take everything so earnestly and seriously. ("Think calmly about what you want to say and then try to talk deliberately and carefully.") Another stereotyped reaction is to look upon stuttering as humorous and amusing. It is often the case, especially among children, that this leads to playful teasing, which, unfortunately, can hurt the stutterer deeply. Comedians who indulge in humor about stuttering also contribute to this. Adult stutterers report that many people often endeavor ineffectively to avoid continuation of the conversation. Frequently, they will try (out of compassion) to continue the stutterer's speech for him or her. In many cases they resort to a conspicuous "sign language" so that the stutterer cannot correctly understand the normal talker. Finally, conversations are abruptly terminated with suggestions to continue the oral interchange in writing.

Stutterers very well know the prejudices and helplessness they engender. They are surprisingly able to predict the magnitude of their speech disorder in a communication situation in which they will participate (Sheehan, 1970c). They know they will not be able to live up to a substantial portion of the rules, norms, and expectations. And it is for just this reason that many of the conventional ritualistic forms of appropriate communication and civility are exceptionally difficult for them. As a result, as adults stutterers have other fixed and complex tendencies. These will be briefly summarized in order to contribute to a better understanding of the following chapter.

Stutterers are hardly in a position to describe exactly the motor-physiological aspect of their stuttering. If they are called upon to signal the precise instant of their stuttering (for example, by raising the hand at the onset of a block) the signal seldom coincides with the objectively determined point because of their very conscious awareness of that moment in their speech. Precise self-awareness and self-description are for the most part possible only after lengthy training and painstaking guidance. It almost appears that as capacity for self-awareness at the moment of a seizure of stuttering does not function there ensue strong feelings of helplessness and powerlessness (Van Riper, 1971).

There are other striking fears that lead to the experience of helplessness in speaking situations. Stutterers generally refuse to listen to themselves on a tape recorder, to talk in front of a mirror, or to permit video recording. Attempts by therapists to record behavior on magnetic tape usually fail, and such activities, should they be necessary for therapeutic measures or diagnostic purposes, are often consequently boycotted by the client (Shearer, 1961). If they do take place the stutterer refuses to listen to or look at the tapes if not required to do so. Only gradual and painstaking effort can accomplish the breakdown of this extreme avoidance behavior and lead to a greater willingness for self-scrutiny. Without doubt the described cognitive loss of control that operates on the tendencies to avoid self-awareness and speech management exerts a strong influence on the subjective rating of competence with which the stutterer enters into a speech situation. This is supported by a large number of investigations dealing with the self-concept of stuttering (especially Freund, 1935; Douglas & Quarrington, 1952; Sheehan, 1954; Buscaglia, 1963; Rieber, 1963).

Consequently, stutterers take on and accept the role of a person who is hardly in a position to establish new contacts. If they do seek attachment to an established group it is usually through the requested intervention of friends or acquaintances. They "let themselves be taken by the hand," let others speak for them, ask others to be helpful in developing friendships. At the same time, stutterers also experiment, and constantly and persistently seek new paths in their quest for new forms of speech. Unfortunately, they lack yardsticks for the assessment of their own performance since they have no experience in what is appropriate and important for communication. Social feedback is withheld from the stutterer out of a false sense of sympathy.

The stutterer takes on the social role that has been assigned to him or her by the caretaker. If he or she does speak just about normally and spontaneously (or right after therapy) face to face with close acquaintances and friends it is not immediately accepted by the parent. Such a situation results in a sense of indignation and unease because the conventional behavior of the interlocutor suddenly ceases. Thus, stutterers report that they are actually happy to stutter again and by reversion they ultimately overcome these periods of illusory freedom from symptoms (Van Riper, 1971).

In summary, we can state that social difficulties have a powerful effect on the cognitive-emotional experience of stutterers. They determine the pattern that the stutterers have designed for themselves and their social position. Cognitive self-concept as it relates to the occurrence of symptoms in a social context derives from socially mediated conduct and attitudes, apprehensions, expectancies, and demands of the environment. Without doubt such cognitive structural variables have behavior-controlling functions in the same way, for example, as contingencies serve as reinforcers of behavior (Fiedler, 1975). These will be treated in more detail in the following section.

COGNITIVE-SOCIAL ASPECTS OF STUTTERING

We have already shown that the functional behavior theory (classical and operant conditioning model) soon approaches its limits when confronted by the complex social determinants of behavior. As a rule, attempts to determine the conjoint responsibility of social-normative conditions for stuttering behavior employ two different analytic strategies. (1) In one of these the attempt is made to describe stuttering as a consequence of *private* awareness processes and cognitively structured stipulations. This notion encompasses theories that place stuttering in the center of internal psychic conflict. Speech disturbances are viewed as the inability of the stutterer to react appropriately to persistently ambivalent conditions. (2) The other theories stress the *social* nature of such conflicts more emphatically and therefore focus on the totality of multifaceted social factors related to stuttering.

In the middle of these two points of view lie the bases of conflicting social stimuli. The first seeks to examine these conflicts as they derive from the *distinctive* cognitive organization of the stutterer as related to social awareness, information processing, and the way in which this organization regulates activity. The conflicts are usually based on the concepts of general psychology and personality theory. The latter are much more strongly oriented to the impact of social structure, the world of norms and standards that pervade the life of the stutterer.

In the preceding section we discussed the many possible situations for generation of social conflict. How they are perceived and cognitively processed by the stutterer are indeed crucial. Here it is possible to think of intrapersonal conflicts that can still be scrutinized as subjective reflection of social and interpersonal conflicts. As such they can express either objective social reality or represent a subjective interpretation as conflict in what are in fact conflict-free social and interpersonal situations.

Intrapersonal Bases of Conflict: Stuttering or Silence?

The speech behavior of stutterers generates a wide variety of social responses. These behaviors entail alternatives among which it is just about impossible or very difficult to choose. The stutterer is more or less constantly in a conflict between talking and not talking as well as between remaining silent or not silent. Most social situations require speech participation by the interacting person and, consequently, also by the stutterer. When he or she talks a social response is called for. Simultaneously, however, the danger of talking leading to a speech disturbance is increased. Moreover, the greater the subjectively experienced responsibility for communication and the greater the situational contingency to talk as normally as possible the more likely will there be a desire to remain silent. Silence removes the danger of the stutterer to attract attention as a "stutterer." But at the same time he or she does not keep up with social requirements and/or accommodate his or her own desire to participate in communication.

Sheehan (1953, 1958) has attempted to portray stuttering as a result of such ambivalence conflicts based on the model of conflict of Miller (1951; also Dollard & Miller, 1950). The devastating operation of the approach-avoidance conflict is that its very nature precludes escape; for withdrawal itself, flight from social situations, is rarely a solution, the more so when it opens up new areas of conflict. Likewise, the only way out of social isolation is again only by communication.

The Cognitive Structure of Intrapersonal Conflicts

The conflict model of Miller is shown in Figure 3-1 displaying approach-avoidance gradients. They are both represented in terms of increasing tendencies of activity toward goals, one to approach a goal (positive valence), one to avoid it (negative valence). However, the avoidance tendency grows more rapidly, that is, the avoidance gradient is steeper.

Miller claims that both tendencies are a function of underlying drive strength (hunger, thirst, inquisitiveness, etc.) and the frequency of their affirmation (which, in fact, functionally determine the nature of approach-avoidance behavior). Thus, drive and social experience determine the strength of the conflict.

It is repeatedly assumed that stutterers usually begin to stutter when the tendency to talk and the tendency to remain silent (cognitive) are equally weighted. These ambitendencies mark the center of the conflict, the point in the diagram where both gradients cross. Hence, stuttering is understood to be a result of the mental tendency to talk or to remain silent wavering around the point of equal valence.

NEUROPSYCHOLOGICAL ASPECTS OF CONFLICT

There are a number of well-known psychophysiological manifestations that are associated with intrapersonal conflict. When resolution of conflict

Figure 3-1 Diagram of Conflict between Approach Tendency (Talking) and Avoidance Tendency (Silence)

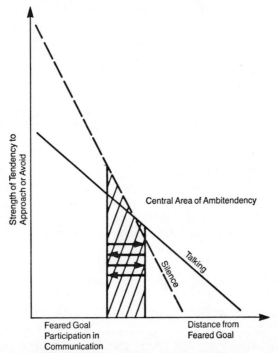

In the central area of conflict, behavior (ambitendency) wavers between talking and silence, leading to stuttering.

is cognitively difficult an excitatory process ensues in the involved person which is reflected in changes in pulse, heartbeat, and blood pressure; in vasoconstriction; in lowering of skin resistance, and in other autonomic reactions. If the conflict resists intrapersonal solution, continuous wavering around the central area of conflict, then habituation to counter the conditions that sustain conflict is prevented (Birbaumer, 1975). The increased state of excitation persists through the experience of helplessness in arriving at a decision. The result is continued inability to cope with the situation. This leads to a condition of anxiety, associated with talking in the case of stuttering, and to other behavioral symptoms that follow the basic principles of classical conditioning. Anxieties again intensify the subjective significance of the conflict and this in turn increases the pressure to decide. The stutterer may react inadequately and impetuously in order to break out of the conflict. Much of the conspicuous mannerisms and habitual social maladjustments of stutterers can be explained by this (note Hostility and Aggression, Krugman, 1946; Santostefano, 1960; Perkins & Haugen, 1971). Unresolvable conflicts lead to a weighty burden ("stress"), out of which additional psychic disturbance can easily develop (Tunner, 1976).

THE ORIGIN OF CONFLICT AND DEVELOPMENT OF STUTTERING

There are particular theories of depth psychology according to which conditions of intrapersonal conflict are considered to be fundamental determinants of stuttering (e.g., Coriat, 1931; Fenichel, 1945; Schneider, 1953; Ockel, 1959; Glauber, 1958; summary, Hofmann, Oertle, & Reincke, 1975; detailed exposition, Orthmann & Scholz, 1975). Schneider (1953) traces stuttering back to unresolved (unknown) conflicts that, triggered in the "instinctive" subconscious, become real in circumstances of excitement and anxiety. Consequently, the "antagonisms in motivation of volition" (e.g., the need to talk, the compulsion to silence) can give rise "to impulses in antagonistic muscles which can evoke tension (spasm)" (p. 18).

For most depth psychologists stuttering is the "encroachment" of an emotional (originating in conflict) disturbance on the physical. Even if the distinctiveness and the inability to validate the assumptions of the depth psychologists have been subjected, in part, to vehement criticism, it appears that their descriptions and observations concerning many conditions of conflict in stutterers are fairly plausible. Thus, the origin of stuttering is seen as a consequence of the unclear rearing practices of the parents, especially as they intervene in the critical period of the development of the child during which he or she passes rapidly through substantial development of striving for independence. The conflicts that lead to stuttering originate in the rearing practices of parents that mitigate against the necessity to arrive at a point in time when these should have long been overcome. However, the practices persist or they reoccur and then interfere with the evolving conventional demands on their development by the intellectual world about them. The "ego" of the child defends itself against these demands and will not let them penetrate the surface, that is, express them. Defense mechanisms are still insufficiently developed and thus the conflicts are revealed. When, for example, the child is expected to talk although he or she really wants to avoid doing so, physical counterreactions (articulatory spasms) result (Glauber, 1958). Anxieties that derive from first arguments with parents gradually evolve into a fear of talking and this produces a continuing degradation of speech. New conditions of conflict emerge since speech is a necessary medium for interpersonal exchange. Children become aware that speech can trigger a reaction from the world about them. To speak a word is synonymous with getting someone to be concerned about them, or, also, just to express joy, rapture, and affection (Barbara, 1954; Glauber, 1958).

With the increase in speech difficulties the child intensifies the struggle against stuttering symptoms. The stutterer is unwilling to put up with his or her helplessness, his or her handicap, or his or her powerlessness. The need when "stuttering" to protect ego gives rise to self-defending processes" (Murphy & Fitzsimons, 1960, p. 171).

Many explanations derived from depth psychology view stuttering symptoms as indications of more causal conflicts and anxieties. Current experiences of conflict that are development dependent lie at the basis of stuttering. In the immediate presence of conflict these result from a great number (that is, affective-cognitive-social) of predisposing determinants.

This brief survey of several points of view of depth psychology should suffice for our purpose. More detailed expositions are to be found in Schilling (1965), Dührssen (1971), Glauber (1958), and Schultheis (1971). The secondary features of neuroses are stressed, for example, by Fernau-Horn (1969). We have filtered out those assessments which, in our opinion, are important and are predominantly addressed to consideration of the origin of conflict. In general, the heterogeneous and thoroughly contradictory theories of stuttering based on depth psychology leave the reader with only a blurred image (Van Riper, 1971; Hofmann, Oertle, & Reincke, 1975). Uneasiness about a psychoanalytic interpretation of stuttering is evident in the work of adherents of depth psychology. Note the views of Freund (1935) and Murphy and Fitzsimons (1960), who sought to combine psychoanalytic points of view with a number of those growing out of learning theories. In the following section we shall refer briefly to one of these based on the work of Sheehan (1970a).

THE SOCIAL ROLE OF THE STUTTERER AND ITS PREDISPOSITION TO CONFLICT

For Sheehan, too, stuttering symptoms are a sign of deep-seated conflict and anxiety (1970c). Nevertheless, he makes it clear that it is not necessary to descend to the "mystical depths," as psychoanalysts do, to find adequate explanations for stuttering (and with it therapeutic help). Rather, Sheehan resorts to the analogy of the iceberg the greatest portion of which lies under the surface (he does not apply the concept "subconscious" to this; he calls this area "private," p. 13). In this domain he localizes all the affective and cognitive aspects of behavior that are due to the anticipation of failure, the expectation of conflict. These conflicts result from manifold experiences of stuttering (and also not stuttering) in socially demanding situations. For Sheehan stuttering is a "subconscious" means to avoid competing efforts (talk–not talk; silence–not silence) because for the client they yield failure.

Sheehan identifies (private) internal sensory as well as psychic feedback processes as contributing to intensification of conflict: (1) impatience of the listener increases the uneasiness of the stutterer; (2) during the immediate speech disturbance the stutterer concentrates on his or her "battle" with speech; (3) this leads to typical focusing on self-control of speech, which leads to further "disregulation" of its satisfactory control.

Sheehan designates this a disturbance of the social representation of "self." Stuttering is a problem of identity. Every stutterer knows both social roles, that of the stutterer and that of the normal talker. In the social role the more distant he or she is from the conflict-burdened self the more he or she can talk fluently (for example, in acting, singing in a choir). Those situations in which disclosure of "self" and its weaknesses are feared are avoided. The behavior and the speech disturbances are to a great extent dependent on the relative status the stutterer occupies in a talking situation (or believes he or she occupies).

These judgments have considerable consequences for therapy. Not training in new ways of talking (symptom therapy) but the attitude of stutterers toward their speech, toward the circumstances of talking and interlocutors, toward their social role—the therapeutic task of self-concept of the stutterer—is central. The stutterer is guided to an intensive analysis of the intrapersonal and social areas of conflict that are at the basis of his or her speech disturbance. The goal is to acquire fresh concepts of the internal and external determinants of stuttering and their firsthand validation in social interaction (in role playing, in therapy groups, etc.). In order to break out of their current role stutterers must know them clearly. In order to overcome their anxieties and fears it is essential for stutterers constantly to seek out social situations fraught with conflict and actively come to an understanding of them. Anxiety and uncertainty persist if new experiences are avoided.

SUMMARY

In this chapter we limited our comment to the most pertinent psychological explanations of stuttering. From our examination of the relevant literature a distinct impression of diversity and heterogeneity of points of view emerges. In the quest for integration most authors dispose of diverse hypotheses with the argument that they are incompatible. The basis for this may well be that it is simpler to evaluate one's own theoretical position (derived understandably from one's own scientific setting) in order to produce an explanatory, diagnostic, and therapeutic corpus therefrom. One associates oneself with one of the traditional or modern "schools" and passes judgment on explanatory efforts and findings of "others" according to whether or not they contribute to the support of one's own position. If not criticized, they are embraced from one's own point of view, or not even referred to.

In this chapter we have left out of consideration many efforts to establish "merit of point of view" and "criticisms" thereof. In the light of current limited knowledge about the development and maintenance of stuttering, these theories turn out to be reciprocal and, in our opinion, lead very definitely to the dead end of theoretical stagnation. When investigations are carried out to support one's own point of view they inevitably lead to the limits of that system and not to basic changes. They rarely suggest the obvious need for theoretical elaboration of their position. Rather, they remain fixed at a point of global conception of a "miniature system," which often attracts an "inflationary boom" of isolated investigations. It is likely that studies are carried out in a manner to minimize the risk of conspicuous failure. They therefore resort to assertions of "theoretical explications of small advances" in very specific (often only experimental) situations (Foppa, 1965).

If we have here avoided continuing discussion of controversial points of view, we have done so with the intention of seeking guidelines to integration. We shall summarize and elaborate them in more detail in the next chapter. The following points summarize our overview of the psychological bases of stuttering:

- Generally, continuing development of the speech disturbance originates in the speech development phase (or it is associated with it—
the so-called *continuity hypothesis*).

- It is further claimed that the transition to stuttering is determined by
contigencies applied by the authorized caretaker, the parent, to the
behavior of the child in the early phases of learning to talk. Of central
importance for the explanation of the development of stuttering is
how parents attend to the child's speech development, what kind of
speech they (consciously or unconsciously) demand, interrupt, reinforce, or punish (Shames).

- Attempts by parents to correct speech or to call attention to it (diagnostic or evaluative), generate and increase problems (Johnson).

- Set demands by parents for better speech and punishment lead to
speech anxieties, which also operate to stabilize symptoms; early
childhood stuttering is a motor expression of somatic and subjective
anxiety (Brutten and Shoemaker, Mowrer).

- Development of a consciousness of stuttering—to be a stutterer and
hardly ever to be able to combat it on one's own—leads to subjective
adjustments and expectancies and in certain social situations inevitably and helplessly to resignation to the disorder (and with it to
failure) (Bloodstein).

- In the course of his or her disturbance, expectancies and anxieties
cause the stutterer to avoid social interaction more and more (Mowrer,
Bloodstein).

- The stutterer finds himself or herself in a conflict between the need to
talk and the fear of social failure (Sheehan).

- Intrapersonal conflicts lead to communicative helplessness and to the
avoidance of social contact; the gravity of the conflict is governed by
the subjectively experienced responsibility for communication in actual
speech situations (self-concept and understanding of role) (Sheehan).

- Conflicts that cannot be resolved generally lead to emotional burdens
that can easily develop into additional psychic aberrations.

In our opinion, the sketch of psychological theories concerned with the
development and maintenance of stuttering reveals a picture of common
and *complementary* features. There are frequent overlappings and similarities in rationales. Still lacking is a satisfactory explanation of conditions
of origin. The reply to questions of the *When* (*status nascendi*) and of the
Why of origin (causal mechanisms) is fixed on a social-psychological level.
Of course, neurophysiological determinants are postulated but in a crude

"somehow or other way" without further delineation. Therefore, it would be interesting to compare the genetic and somatic hypotheses/perceptions presented in Chapter 2 with the psychological thinking described in this chapter to see if there is the possibility of a common explanation for the pathogenesis of stuttering. We shall do this in the following chapter.

Chapter 4

The Search for Integration: Stuttering as a Neuropsychological Phenomenon

INTRODUCTION

The manifold psychological and medical attempts to explain stuttering are so confounding that it is hazardous to attempt a synthesis. Nevertheless, we shall try to reconcile somatic and psychological theories. In explaining the phenomenon of stuttering until now it has become clear that separation of neurophysiological/neuromuscular mechanisms from psychological processes is not at all profitable. It can be confidently asserted that at the basis of every stutter reaction there are physiologic-motor as well as social-cognitive (causal) conditions involving interindividual and intraindividual aspects involved inseparably in distinctive ways with one another. The frequently advanced distinction between "innate" and "learned" contributions to stuttering does not entirely enlighten us as to its origin. For our purposes three helpful statements representing a synopsis of previous chapters are in order:

1. Somatic views are appropriate for explanation of the *origin* and *cause* of stuttering.
2. Attempts at psychological explanations are largely applied to understanding the *development* and *maintenance* of stuttering.
3. Attempts at integration should take into account the interaction between constitutional and psychological factors.

We shall treat our subject in two parts. In the first we shall undertake integration of diverse ideas. A point of departure for this will be the evident interrelations between physiological and psychological, innate and learned, aspects of the stuttering syndrome (in this chapter). In the next part we present an integrative model of an overall scheme for diagnosis and behavior modification of stuttering (Figure 4-1). This model should contribute to the classification, evaluation, and organization of diagnostic data and then can be applied, as such, to the formulation of individualized plans for therapy and for their implementation and supervision (in Chapter 5).

A NEUROPSYCHOLOGICAL MODEL OF THE ORIGIN AND MAINTENANCE OF STUTTERING

Even with a semblance of validity it is currently impossible to describe the neurophysiological processes involved in speech development. Cybernetic approaches, too, have their limitations in formulating the issues in terms of systems theory. Our intent here is the design of a global neuropsychological model of the interrelations having to do with the causality of stuttering that would enable gross integration of well-known phenomena. In making our case for integration we shall necessarily have to speculate about the field. Furthermore, we shall avoid any pretension to completeness.

INTERFERENCES WITH AUDITORY FEEDBACK AND "NORMAL" SPEECH DISTURBANCE

With rare exceptions the development of conspicuous symptoms of stuttering takes place gradually and largely rather imperceptibly. As we have seen, children from the ages of 2 to 4 generally go through a phase of "developmental stuttering." Conspicuous word and syllable repetitions resemble the descriptions of stuttering symptoms noted in Chapter 1 only remotely. Most authors consider that this "normal" stuttering constitutes the onset of the development of speech disturbance. Exceptions with later onset of speech difficulties are almost universally linked with external influences and causes (Chapter 2).

Van Riper (1971) has presented a plausible explanation of the phenomenon of "developmental stuttering" based on the theory of auditory control of speech, which we incorporate in our global neuropsychological model shown in Figure 4-1 (see also Widlak & Fiedler, 1977). The central element of the model is the coordination of speech production. The assumed unity of the central nervous system regulates via the motor system the intensity and duration of signals generated by the speech musculature (output coordination). The unity of the sensory system is responsible for all incoming information that is essential for coordinated sequencing of speech (input coordination). As we have seen, incoming information constitutes the fundamental stimuli produced by one's own speech that "report

Figure 4-1 Neuropsychological Model of Gross Influences on Self-Control of Speech

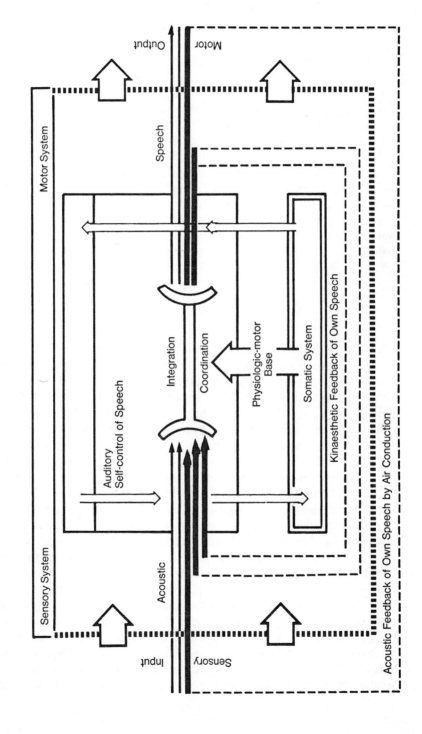

back" over air, bone, and kinesthetic pathways of the integrative-coordinating system.

Since these multiple signals require significantly different speeds of transmission over the individual channels/neural pathways, they arrive at the control center at considerably different times. It is easy to see that different kinds of disturbances can result from the variety of feedback channels as well as from the many signals that are fed back which in turn greatly impair proper coordination of speech. From this we proceed in our model to the assumption that stuttering can ensue because varying speeds of conduction of fed back speech signals in the integrative-coordinating system interfere with one another to such an extent that they can no longer be integrated neurophysiologically. Coordination of speech is disturbed. Control of the speech act is not possible or it is marked by disturbance. Similar speech disturbances can also be produced in normal-speaking individuals when, for instance, their own utterances are transmitted to them over headphones with a short time delay (Lee Effect, Chapter 2).

DEVELOPMENTAL STUTTERING

How then does "normal" developmental stuttering occur during the period of speech development? We can assume that during the phase of speech learning (sounds and syllables) the fundamental instrument of speech control by the child is largely auditory feedback. In the course of speech development control function of the speech apparatus is increasingly taken over by surface sensitivity (touch and contact) and by deeper sensitivity (position and movement). Auditory channels are used for reception of external stimuli; they are increasingly reserved for "intellectual" control of private and social determinants of behavior.

In this transition to control of speech by kinesthetic feedback there are usually disturbing interferences if auditory feedback operates along with the kinesthetic. They result from time differences and phase shifts among the diverse feedback signals the precise structure of which is not yet known (see Chapter 2). If the interfering feedback signals cannot be integrated, orderly coordination of the muscle groups contributing to the speech act is impeded. Presumably, as a result of the failure of integration, the cortically controlled innervation of the speech musculature is no longer or hardly sufficiently synchronized. The child stutters because a desynchronization of impulses guiding central programming of muscle groups leads to masking of impulses and/or their interruption (Chapter 2). Thus, the mild to severe speech disturbances of developmental stuttering can be explained as a desynchronized coordination of the speech sequence the cause of which lies in the defect of integration of interfering feedback signals from vocal output.

RETENTION OF AUDITORY SPEECH CONTROL AND SYMPTOMATIC STUTTERING

Normal speech is controlled primarily by the surface and deep sensitivities of the speech mechanism. This can be observed strikingly in stutterers themselves. If the normal acoustic feedback is masked out by white noise, a reduction or complete disappearance of the speech disturbance is observed, depending on the intensity of the noise (also in those with a long history of symptoms) (Chapter 2). If the stutterer controls his or her speech exclusively by kinesthesia, the symptoms disappear almost completely. Since this is a well-known phenomenon in adult stuttering, it follows that impairing influences similar to the ones we have postulated for developmental stuttering are at the basis of the speech disturbances, disturbances that derive from interferences of auditory feedback and of coordination of speech.

The assumptions of the model suggest a neurophysiological (constitutional) cause of stuttering. Yet there are always situations in which stutterers speak fluently; to name a few, when talking to themselves or with individuals who are well acquainted with them or whom they know well. Time and again this observation is used to argue against the assumption of a neurophysiological cause. Does it really contradict this assumption?

In the transitional phase from auditory to kinesthetic control of speech production, interruptions and excessive rapidity of the flow of speech occur for most children, which we label normal developmental stuttering. If during this period speech disfluencies are noted by the relevant caretaker (parent), corrected, or even punished, it is likely that the child intensifies his or her efforts to improve speech. The child will "revert" to exclusive auditory control of speech and will "listen to himself or herself" in an effort to improve production of poorly spoken words and sentence fragments. Thus the auditory feedback channel retains its significance for control of speech output.

With the continuing development of speech there is a constantly increasing need to control the contextual continuity of spoken sentences and passages. To facilitate this the auditory mode is increasingly used for contact with, and control of, the milieu, as for instance, in direct reception and processing of social feedback. It is probable that in doing this the control of speech by kinesthetic feedback *must* be instituted to a substantial degree, in order to free the auditory pathway for tasks requiring "intellectual" control.

During this period the outside world (parents, rearers) then sets up significant contingencies that are associated less with substantive and considerably more with qualitative features of speech (its excellence). Thus auditory control of speech is "forced" on the talker. If there is a simultaneous increase in speech control by kinesthetically fed back impulses, an increase in impairing interferences follows and stuttering ensues. This suggests the likelihood that stuttering develops from retained auditory control and increasing kinesthetic control of speech. The temporally varying feedback speech signals cannot be integrated and control impulses to the speech musculature cannot be coordinated. Responsible for the "excessive attention" to the acoustic signals of one's own speech are substantial environmental factors, which we shall discuss in somewhat more detail in the following section.

SPEECH TRAINING AND SYMPTOMATIC STUTTERING

Here we ask two questions. First: What environmental factors contribute to the maintenance of auditory control of speech? And for every child who presumably needs a longer time for auditory control of speech output there is the second question: Why do most children stutter for only a short time during the phase of speech development and some probably not at all?

During the period of speech learning the environment (as a rule caretakers such as parents, older siblings, etc.) frequently calls attention to the errors in a child's speech. Assistance and instruction referring to lip positions, breathing techniques, and formation of individual sounds are given. The child acquires speech but imitation, modeling, and demonstration also are likely to be involved. In the process of imitation the child compares his or her own speech with that of the model, and it gets "drilled" until the speech model is simulated. As this takes place auditory control of speech becomes less significant, all the more so as the criterion for similarity or agreement with the selected and previously presented model is satisfied. Usually, the indication for this is that the caretaker no longer pays attention to the quality of speech and does not comment on the adequacy and correctness of joining speech units (words and sentences) or elicit their repetition. The focus is on control of content rather than the quality of what is said.

There is much evidence that coincidental with these environmental signals of assistance, instruction, and modeling, punishment is usually instituted when the quality of speech is hardly or only sluggishly improved. As we pointed out in Chapter 3, caretakers generally react to speech disfluencies with a worried expression, impatience, irritation, and additional reliance on punishment. It is easy to see that such aversive consequences for the child reinforce the subjective need to control his or her own speech acoustically, in order to avoid aversive stimuli (interpreted in learning psychology as escape behavior). Or the consequences are avoided in the first place by auditory self-control of speech (avoidance behavior). It follows from this that the cause of maintenance of auditory control by the child is to be sought primarily in the continuing attention to quality of speech and its control in response to environmental circumstances. Simultaneous increase in kinesthetic control of speech, a necessary condition for freeing the auditory channel for concentration on the content of speech and for continued attention to the environment, leads to stuttering brought on by interferences in feedback channels.

Now to the second question: Why does the phase of "normal" environmental stuttering pass uneventfully for most children? It is conceivable that during this rapid period of speech development the caretaker reinforces attention to the essence of speech (vocabulary, word sequence, sentence structure, and the message itself), facilitated by the transition to kinesthetic control of speech output. In this process auditory control is probably still used sporadically, for instance, for production of certain complicated words. Thus, it is likely that before long the child achieves correct production, i.e., *proper* kinesthetic control. With the establishment of the kinesthetic feedback code and with the programming of coordinated neuromotor flow of speech, the importance of auditory control of speech fades quickly. Problems (i.e., stuttering symptoms) obviously persist only if the various feedback channels maintain their equivalence in controlling speech output. Studies of Webster's research group (1968, 1970; Chapter 2) suggest that in normal-speaking individuals elevation of the threshold of awareness of the acoustic signal produced by one's own voice accompanies increasing central attention to the social and content aspects of communication. It may be that in stutterers the threshold of awareness of one's own voice remains depressed as a result of constant drilling on auditory self-control. If the threshold remains depressed, interferences among various feedback channels become prominent and integration becomes difficult.

HEREDITY AND STUTTERING

From research on twins and the frequent occurrence of stuttering in certain families, as well as the uneven distribution according to sex (recall that four times as many boys stutter as girls), we cannot rule out with certainty that the assumption of a hereditary component for stuttering is unwarranted (Chapter 2). Without going into extensive speculation on the particular hereditary factors bearing on stuttering, the point needs to be made that the auditory interferences can be attributed in part to inherited neurophysiological conditions. We can deduce from several of the investigations cited in Chapter 2 that probably there are greater constitutionally determined discrepancies in males in the transmission time of feedback signals. Studies of delayed feedback of speech indicate that females adapt better, i.e., learn more rapidly, to speak without error under conditions of contrived auditory interferences.

In the course of normal development of speech, as we have surmised, the threshold of awareness of the acoustic signal in one's own speech is apparently elevated; in stutterers it remains manifestly depressed. These findings also suggest that there is a prominent hereditary causal concomitant of stuttering. Hence, there is a congenitally depressed threshold for the acoustic signals of one's own speech. We suspect, however, an interaction between physiological and psychological factors. Constant subjectively experienced demands of the environment for an improving quality of speech result in a continuous subjective need for auditory control of one's own speech. Training causes the threshold to remain depressed. It may also be that genetic predispositions may stand in the way of threshold elevation (Chapter 2).

The conditions that have been described here can also be considered to contribute to an explanation and prognosis of spontaneous remission. Comparatively depressed threshold values for the acoustic signal of one's own speech presumably make   adaptation always more difficult and so spontaneous remission of stuttering becomes more improbable the more sensitive the auditory awareness of one's own speech becomes.

THE MAINTENANCE OF STUTTERING AND SUBJECTIVELY EXPERIENCED RESPONSIBILITY FOR COMMUNICATION

Arguments previously presented support rather substantially the thesis of situation dependency of stuttering and that indeed it is one of its most prominent signs. We have expressed this idea in our model (Figure 4-1) in introducing subjectively experienced responsibility for communication of the stutterer as an essential variable. This constitutes a cognitive basis for excessive attention to auditory control of speech. If it diminishes, then conspicuous stuttering symptoms usually diminish. As we have said before, there are a number of situations in which responsibility for communication is reduced. Stuttering symptoms are reduced in adult clients with longer histories of symptoms when they sing in a choir and when they speak alone or with children. These are social situations that are subjectively unburdensome and in which qualitatively perfect speech is not called for unconditionally. However, with a surge of subjectively experienced accountability for communication there is a drastic increase in symptoms (in the presence of certain persons, in crucially demanding situations). It is the number of symptoms, not their loci, that increases. It is always the same or similar word units, sounds, or places in a sentence that characterize the stuttering (consistency effect; Chapter 1). Here the following complementary point needs to be made. The utterance of the stutterer is subjectively concentrated particularly on those sounds and sound sequences that are considered by him or her to be especially prone to disturbance. Any stutterer can state precisely which sounds and syllables, vowels and consonants give rise to special difficulties and he or she is likely to "attend" to them more intensely.

Our model also incorporates the adaptation effect (Chapter 1). This is based on the spontaneous buildup of motor speech patterns. An immediate motor speech sequence is programmed, so to speak, an effect that is also noted in normal-speaking individuals who reduce the number of errors on repeated reading of a text. Buildup of motor sets renders control over the auditory feedback channel less prominent and thereby reduces the interferences that lead to interruptions in speech (Widlak & Fiedler, 1977; also Frank & Bloodstein, 1971).

EXTERNAL CONTROL AND FAILURE-FREE SPEECH

A number of other conditions contribute to symptom-free or symptom-reduced speech of the stutterer. One of the most important of these is rhythmic speech. Van Riper (1971) reported that a British physician named Thewall introduced rhythmic speech in the treatment of a stuttering client (also Chapter 6). Johnson and Rosen (1937) carried out an early controlled experiment in which stutterers had the least amount of failures when they spoke words, or their syllables, in rhythmic fashion. Van Dantzig (1940) had stutterers accompany each syllable with finger tapping on the edge of a table, which immediately resulted in fluent speech. More recently a number of studies have been done in which a rhythmic source (for example, a metronome) was introduced with which the stutterer had to keep time while speaking syllables and words (Beech & Fransella, 1971; also Chapter 6).

It is clear that the neurophysiological mechanism responsible for the diminution of stuttering when speech is produced in a variety of rhythms is *not* to be sought exclusively in a desynchronization of the central impulses to the speech musculature. Rather, stuttering originates as a consequence of active feedback interferences. The orientation ("imagined" by the stutterer and/or externally provided) to the rhythmic stimulus permits coordinated motor speech activity! The validity of this proposition is supported by additional observations. As we have seen, there is marked improvement in stutterers under conditions of masking by white noise as well as when auditory feedback is delayed (Chapter 2). In these situations auditory feedback no longer affects coordination of the speech act; the stutterer must coordinate his or her own speech largely without recourse to information about his or her speech fed back over the auditory channel. Kinesthetic information predominates and enables fluent speech.

Normal speech is approximated when the stutterer is instructed to read a text almost simultaneously with another reader (so-called "shadow speech," Cherry & Sayers, 1956; also Chapter 6). We have previously pointed out similar observations of stutterers speaking and singing "along" in choirs. And the stutterer hardly errs when singing aloud by himself or herself. These are conditions under which this communication responsibility in the presence of a listener can be preserved and under which fluent speech can occur. The stutterer presumably coordinates his or her speech (or singing) by orienting to the external stimulus (the speech of the reader) or to the rhythm and melody of the tune. The findings that stutterers can talk with spontaneous fluency in many situations refute the notion of automated failure behavior that over a longer period of time can imbed itself as a full-fledged autonomic "habit." (Thus, Wendlandt, 1972).

A PARADOX: STUTTERING AND THE SUBJECTIVE EFFORT TO IMPROVE SPEECH

If the assumptions of our model are correct then every effort of the stutterer to improve speech produces consolidation of his or her symptoms. The attempt to control stuttering leads to stuttering, a presumption that has already been stated by other authors and even on different theoretical grounds (Johnson, 1956c; Bloodstein, 1958; Wischner, 1952). Because of this apparent impossibility for self-control of speech the stutterer finds himself or herself in a hopeless position. In the face of existing and increasing demands for better speech he or she cannot attain it because the control reactions (mostly auditory self-control of speech) are jointly responsible for the stuttering. This paradoxical situation which the stutterer can no longer overcome constantly stimulates the stutterer to seek ever novel techniques of control. We presume that most of accessory symptoms (associated movements, irregular breathing) served the stutterer very well at the time of initial use. It is simple to explain what follows. If we encourage the stutterer to engage in activity concurrent with speech (as, for example, rhythmic finger tapping, foot stamping, piano playing, and dancing), the stuttering symptoms decrease considerably. In doing this the stutterer concentrates primarily on the new activity whereby conscious auditory monitoring of his or her own speech is reduced. Furthermore, it is clear that concentrated control of motor activity is no longer necessary. Attention can again be directed to other areas. With each minor failure in talking, attention is presumably again focused on speech behavior. The concomitant symptoms remain, probably because their short-term effect is repeated intermittently. They become an established component of the symptom picture.

In further development of the disorder the stutterer very soon recognizes that control of stuttering is beyond reach. He or she feels overtaxed. The constant effort, the persistent recurrence of futile attempts to achieve control, generate experiences and feelings of helplessness, hopelessness, and burden (stress), which are reflected in manifold autonomic and subjective anxieties. This leads to persistent aggravating states and autonomic stress reactions (so-called "general activation syndrome," Birbaumer, 1975), which can result in psychosomatic illnesses.

The paradox that has been described also presents a therapeutic dilemma. If the stutterer wants to overcome stuttering he or she must not control his or her speech auditorily. However, can this be effectively instituted by the stutterer? How difficult it is for the stutterer to abandon efforts at self-monitoring is demonstrated in therapeutic views that a stutterer must be guided at the outset to complete acceptance of his or her disorder. Thus, the self-control of speech as a goal will thereby lose its essence and purpose and, therefore, its symptom-stabilizing function (Sheehan, 1970d). These approaches suggest that they are the path to a lasting result. They confront their limits when social circumstances mitigate against acceptance (or minimizing) of symptoms. Already during the period of speech development, as we have seen, caretakers make great demands for good speech production. Parents themselves are under social pressure and are responsible for the intellectual and behavioral growth of their children. It is difficult for them to tolerate stuttering. Rather, they do all they can to "help" the child overcome speech difficulties. In many cases exhortations (all of this largely without an awareness of the inevitable consequences) carry over to a worrisome concern for good speech and this leads to maintenance of developmental stuttering.

In our model there is also evidence for the correctness of Johnson's views (1956a) that stuttering is a result of its diagnosis (Chapter 3). Frequent demand for the earliest possible recognition of disorder (for example, to expect favorable prognosis due to proper management in childhood) appears to be extremely questionable in the light of observed symptom development. The most practical recommended strategy during that time is not to look for stuttering symptoms but to tolerate them (recommendations by Johnson and many other authors). We shall return to this point when we discuss preventive measures in detail (Chapter 10).

COGNITIVE-SOCIAL DETERMINANTS OF STUTTERING

Our previous reference to expected parental reactions was clearly limited to consideration of intrapersonal causal conditions. The construct "subjectively experienced communication responsibility" incorporates social determinants. Our model shows close dependency of the origin and course of stuttering symptoms on positive and negative influences of the social milieu. The source and genesis of the speech disorder are tied directly to conditions of the interpersonal and social setting. Children become stutterers by way of the conditions of their social world that control their language and their learning of speech. Adult stutterers, too, can and must be seen in relation to social context. It follows that the demands on adults for perfect speech as compared with children are much more intense, the more so if their occupations include a need for speech. There is a great deal of evidence that stutterers are confronted by prejudice and obstacles not only in their immediate social environment but also continue to be denied advancement and improvement in social status as well as many other social privileges because of their speech disorder.

The actual social conditions responsible for the intensification or reduction of subjectively experienced communication responsibility of stutterers are manifold and complex. They are not exclusively revealed by painstaking analysis of the inner evaluating systems of the stutterer, although this affords very important points of contact. They are largely determined by the stutterer's personal evaluations of experiences (learning experiences) in relating to communication situations involving actual experience and activity (talking). The assessment of a speech situation as more or less threatening, as difficult or easy, as important or unimportant, leads to expectations (anticipations) as to whether and how an actual impending exchange will be controlled. Outcomes and failures that have been experienced in the past enter into assessments and anticipations and determine the stutterer's subjective prediction about his or her real social competence.

In the context of diverse social situations the stutterer himself or herself largely determines how intensified (or depressed) his or her communication responsibility is and thereby his or her communication competence. It is the cognitive self-concept and the cognitive concept of the situation that determine the degree of disturbances. The high prognostic value of self-appraisal of speech disturbances in given contexts is evidence for this (Chapter 3). However, whether these self-concepts of the stutterer reflect real conditions accurately or just "refract" them can be settled by examining those circumstances wherein the stutterer seeks company and conversation with other people or avoids them. In every case these social and cognitive determinants must be taken into account in diagnosis and therapy.

The relatively negligible results of stuttering therapy may perhaps be attributed to concentration on improvement of disordered speech and to neglect of the cognitive-social aspects of the problem. From this standpoint, temporary placement in a facility for speech therapy is questionable. If the individual who has been so managed returns to his or her former living situation when (more or less effective) therapy has been terminated the necessary variety of conditions for symptom-free speech is lacking. The foremost of these is subjectively experienced communication responsibility. For the most part this is aggravated by parents' expectations (justifiably?) from the intramural treatment. The self-control of efforts to improve speech exclusively is reinforced. All of this calls into question the continuation of laboriously acquired behavioral changes as the aim of therapy.

Our model clearly rejects speech-only therapy. Rather, therapeutic intervention must also address the everyday real-life behavior of the stutterer. In so doing diagnostics and planning for therapy make sufficient allowance for social determinants. Along with attention to aspects of intrapersonal behavior a behavioral analysis of stuttering must conscientiously strive for a clarification of interpersonal and social conditions that indicate the degree of subjectively experienced communication responsibility of the stutterer. Then it is likely that therapy for stuttering will attain its desired goal if it accommodates the mutual cognitive and social determinants as they have been briefly set forth here.

SUMMARY

In explaining the phenomena of stuttering this chapter has endeavored to narrow the distance between neurophysiological/neuromuscular mechanisms on the one hand and psychological factors on the other. Physiological-motor as well as social-cognitive (causal) conditions underlie stutter reaction. Therefore, the view that stuttering is a neurophysiological phenomenon only is rejected. How these conditions interweave with one another is not entirely clear. This explains the global and largely speculative character of the ideas of the proposed model.

We proceed with the premise that the proposition that auditory feedback interferences are a cause of normal speech disturbances of early childhood is open to question. The probability has been suggested that symptomatic stuttering develops from the retention of auditory self-control of speech (and incidentally the continuing feedback interferences). However, vital environmental factors also appear to be responsible for this. Central to our proposed hypotheses is the cognitive aspect of the stutterer's responsibility for communication. Intensely experienced communication responsibility results in anxious self-control of speech, which in turn leads to feedback interferences and finally to severe discoordination of speech. Stuttering ensues.

This chapter points up the frequently repeated argument that every attempt of the stutterer to improve his or her speech (by auditory self-control of speech) is inevitably doomed to failure. They even provoke difficulties, which in turn generate concomitant symptoms and other disturbances.

The significance which we attach to the cognitive-social aspects of stuttering requires that we devote special attention to their consequences for therapy. In Part II we shall attempt to apply the ideas we have considered up to this point to recommendations for diagnosis and therapy.

Part II

Diagnosis and Therapy for Stuttering

A Diagnostic Schema for Preparation of Therapeutic Measures for the Treatment of Stuttering

INTRODUCTION

Before we proceed to detailed treatment procedures a summary of previous theoretical discussions should constitute a useful transition. However, instead of merely repeating hypotheses and facts we shall try to construct a management framework on the basis of findings that may still be either at issue or perhaps well documented. This should assist the therapist in dealing with the task of moving from the diagnostic to the therapeutic phase. In this chapter we shall present what from our point of view is a system by which information relevant for therapy can be ascertained, evaluated, and interpreted for each individual case.

In a general way we shall fall back on current schema for diagnosis and planning of behavior therapy introduced by Schulte (1974). Schulte's schema recommends itself quite adequately for work with individual cases since it is not only helpful as a framework for collection and organization of information but it is also suitable for determining therapy. This schema should also serve as a useful guideline as we move on to presentation and elucidation of diagnostic-therapeutic decisions. With Schulte's suggested framework as a reference we shall elaborate and put in concrete terms pertinent information about the conditions related to the onset of stuttering. Finally, as suggested in the last two chapters, much more prominent consideration will be given to the cognitive aspects of the diagnostic and therapeutic task. For this we shall adopt recommendations for diagnostic and therapeutic application of cognitive determinants as submitted by Fiedler (1978a).

A summary outline of the schema for diagnosis and therapy is given below:

1. Description of the speech disorder

1.1. Data collection: Balbutiogram
   (1) Speaking sequences
   (2) Sentence repetition
   (3) Reading from a standard text
   (4) Free speech
1.2. Observations of motor-physiological characteristics
   (1) Basic symptomatology
   (2) Oral motor patterns
   (3) Physiological concomitants
1.3. Linguistic characteristics
   (1) Determination of locus
   (2) Semantic characteristics
   (3) Consistency of stuttering
   (4) Adaptation to stuttering
1.4. Concomitant symptoms
1.5. Variability in stuttering
   (1) Whispered reading
   (2) Reading and white noise
   (3) Rhythmic speaking
   (4) Simultaneous speaking
   (5) Varying the situation
1.6. Cognitive aspects of stuttering
   (1) Stimulus assessments
   (2) Assessment of experiences
   (3) Assessment of behavior/expectancies of competence
   (4) Regulation of behavior
1.7. Organic variables
1.8. Genesis of stuttering
   (1) The onset of conspicuous stuttering
   (2) Causal factors
   (3) Development of the disorder
   (4) Rearing characteristics
   (5) Hereditary factors
2. Description of social difficulties and additional conspicuous behaviors
   2.1. Specific conditions
      (1) Description of symptomatic behavior
      (2) Stimulus reactions
      (3) Organic variables
   2.2. Social analysis
3. Differential diagnosis of the boundaries of the speech disorder
   3.1. Stuttering and cluttering

3.2. Stuttering and stammering
3.3. Stuttering and symptomatic iterations
4. Analysis of conditions
    4.1. Determinants of the speech disorder
        (1) Respondent control of behavior
        (2) Operant control of behavior
        (3) Cognitive control of behavior
    4.2. Determinants of social disturbance
        (1) Social models
        (2) Restricted social activity
    4.3. Summary of analysis
        (1) Development of stuttering and social disturbance
        (2) Direct determinants of stuttering and concomitant conspic-
            uous behaviors
5. General considerations for preparing therapeutic measures
    5.1. The need for interdisciplinary decisions
    5.2. The age of the stutterer

If this schema is followed, the diagnostic tasks of the therapist follow sequentially, starting from a very detailed description of the speech disorder, proceeding to an analysis, in a broad sense, of the emotional, cognitive, and social determinants, and leading from there to a summarizing assessment of overall symptomatology. Finally, this model becomes the basis for therapy. In the following chapter we shall return in detail to the choices of therapeutic interventions. We shall next fill in the contents of the schema outline. This will combine material from preceding chapters and relevant appropriate findings.

1. DESCRIPTION OF THE SPEECH DISORDER

In the preceding chapters stuttering has been described as a complex behavioral disturbance at the focus of which are multifaceted interdependent circumstantial variables. In what follows we shall analyze the speech disorder in a restricted sense. Additional personal and situational variables are added piece by piece and are fitted into the configuration that defines the distinctive symptomatology of the individual client. Unlike the basic researcher the therapist comes upon multiple symptom peculiarities developed in the course of time and from these he or she must try by hindsight to identify the conditions that are essentially responsible for or contribute to directing and maintaining the behavior (Schulte, 1974). The weight of the various determinants has to be precisely ascertained so that their relevance to therapy may be firmly established.

Accurate description has another function in addition to preparation for therapy. It serves the therapist as a basis of comparison during the course of and at the termination of treatment which can be used as a referent for possible changes in behavior and which can assist in specifying "outcomes of therapy." Indeed, the more accurately the particular symptoms (qualitative and quantitative) of the client are established at the outset of therapy the more the results of therapy can be specified. Both of these points of view, gathering of information for preparation and planning of therapy as well as use as a data base for specification of changes in symptoms and behavior, need to be kept in mind in accurate completion of the following subsections.

1.1. Data Collection: Balbutiogram

For the following diagnostic steps (as well as later measurement of results) an accurate assessment of speech disorder is recommended. This will involve baselines and failure frequency rates related to basic rates. These and similar measures can be repeated regularly during the course of therapy in order to note changes in speech behavior. For this purpose Lüking proposes the preparation of a so-called balbutiogram, which gives the investigator a record of the frequency of stuttering under varying conditions. This appears to be the most economical procedure in terms of effort and time (1957, 1960; also Böhme, 1977, p. 43f.). Such a balbutiogram is proposed in somewhat modified form in the following four steps, which will later be elaborated as individual measures:

(1) Speaking sequences

The client is asked to continue counting from a particular number and to name the days of the week or months. He or she can also recite a familiar poem, which the therapist can control. Poorly spoken syllables are recorded with a " − " and properly spoken ones with a " +." Failure-free speech can be recorded as " + + + + ...". Measures of repetitions in later sessions should obviously be carried out at the same point.

(2) Sentence repetition

Several short sentences of a text are read out loud or spoken by the therapist and are immediately repeated freely by the client, i.e., without having to imitate precisely. Sentence length is determined by the individual characteristics of the client as the circumstances may require (for example, age, capacity for memory). Here, too, minus marks can be used at the point where stuttering occurs and entered directly in the spaces between lines. Underlining can also be used. In this way it is easy to record the precise locus of the stuttering, which words, at which letters, sounds, and syllables and whether the stuttering was clonic or tonic, etc.

(3) Reading from a standard text

A text should be selected that contains no more than 300 to 400 words and that has the least possible emotional significance for the stutterer. The text lies before the therapist so that entries (in the margins) can be simultaneously recorded. It is helpful if the client agrees to permit sound and/or video recording since this facilitates precise assessment of speech disorders. Analyses of recorded behavior such as these yield several additional measures: total speech time, frequency of stuttering, maximum symptom-free time, word count (for omissions or repeated or inserted words), and eventually duration of stuttering.

(4) Free speech

Free speech usually presents a much greater degree of difficulty than reading. It is much more important for communication and thus is a better criterion for evaluating results of therapy. The client is required to talk on a suggested theme (for example, description of a room or a childhood experience). The themes should ensure that in measuring various repetitions the difficulties are of approximately equal level. A time limit of about 3 or 4 minutes is satisfactory. Similar evaluation of the kind used with the read text (and with sound and video recording) can be applied here.

Such a balbutiogram as well as the tape recordings can help with other overall descriptions:

1.2. Observations of Motor-Physiological Characteristics

The motor defects and characteristics of the stuttering revealed in the balbutiogram should then be organized as follows and provisionally assessed:

(1) Basic symptomatology

Is the symptom picture predominantly clonic (i.e., reoccurring short, sequential, audible repetitions of a syllable, a word, or a sound)?

Or are there tonic signs in the stuttering (as silent or audible prolongations with the onset of articulation)?

Or is it a mixed form where one or the other symptom predominates (clonic-tonic or tonic-clonic)?

(2) Oral motor patterns

In order to have sufficient basis for subsequent measures of change, an accurate description of blocks and hesitations is required:

During speech are there conspicuous spasms of the lips, tongue, mandible, and neck musculature?

If so:

Are the spasms relatively long? Or are they brief contractions following rapidly one after another?

Does the articulatory gesture with which the stutterer attempts a sound correspond to the conventional position of the mouth for that sound?

Is the mouth open or shut during the spasm?

Is there a grinding of teeth?

Are glottal stops audible?

Are spasms or abnormally bizarre movements of the tongue observable?

How do total motor lapses of various stuttering sequences look (for example, in mixed forms)?

In addition, breathing behavior during speech needs to be observed and described.

Is speech produced with inspired or residual air?

When and how does the client take a breath?

Is there gasping for breath during speech?

Are there changes in pitch and rate during speaking of sentences?

(3) Physiological concomitants

When possible inquiry into physiological correlates of speech disorder is indicated:

Is there evenly paced activation of talking? Or is there conspicuous agitation during speech, for example, when there is an "obligation to talk?"

Is secretion of perspiration observable in the face?

If at all possible, can measures of physiological variables such as pulse, blood pressure, psychogalvanic resistance (PGR), and other characteristics be determined during speech?

It should be noted that in this organizational scheme still another precise description of individual symptoms is involved. Data related to situation-dependent stuttering as well as additional data on frequency and oscillations will be taken up more precisely under point 1.5 or as the need for elucidation may be required here.

1.3. Linguistic Characteristics

A second group of observable characteristics of stuttering that may constitute a basis for subsequent therapy and measurement of change is additional marked features that go along with the disorders of speech. Here the distinctive linguistic and semantic peculiarities need to be recorded and organized. Access to these is best accomplished through free discourse.

(1) Determination of locus

Does the stuttering reaction occur largely with consonants or vowels? Which with greater frequency?
Do these words occur at the beginning of sentences or later?
Are they mainly longer or shorter words?
Are certain words or kinds of words exclusively conspicuous?
Are sequences of voiceless and voiced sounds noteworthy?

(2) Semantic characteristics

Semantic devices are usually employed by the stutterer in social interactions in face of the need to speak fluently (Chapter 1). Several interviews at different times are recommended. These reveal how certain marked and regular mannerisms are inserted while talking. These may be organized as follows:

(a) *Embolophones*: Bridging sounds (such as "oh," "ah," "hmm," etc.) as they also occur in normal speech—although less frequently; this also applies to

(b) *Embolophrases*: Bridging words, phraselike parts of sentences, or sentences that are inserted during speech pauses or as beginnings of sentences (such as "shall we say," "I believe," "so to speak," etc.).

(c) *Sentence transposition and word substitution*: We find these in almost all stutterers. Difficult words that are frequently stuttered (for example, "Today it is very --w--w--w, ar-- very hot outside.") are avoided.

(d) *Starters*: Starters are regularly inserted sounds or phrases that are easy to say and are usually inserted at the beginning of an utterance when the pressure of time or other compelling demands of the situation do not allow for delay of speech (for example, "I really think that ----" or "I really don't have much to say about that!"). Generally, starters are spoken fluently.

(e) *Stop-go mechanism*: When the (largely clonic) stutterer has stuttered in articulating a sound, a syllable, or word fragment, he or she starts the articulation over again (for example: "l-u, l-u, l-u ---- love"). Stop-go mechanisms are also used by tonic stutterers (as Hand--t--t----, Handtuch, ah, Handtuch).

(3) Consistency of stuttering

In the diagnostic phase it is generally advisable to collect data on the consistency of stuttering (Chapter 1). This can indicate the severity of the disorder. The stutterer is asked to read a short portion of text several times successively (supplementing the balbutiogram). The frequency with which repetitions occur in the same place in the text determines the consistency (stated as percentages of possibilities in the text). In order to determine the influence of time on the consistency effect it is advisable to include in later sessions repeated readings and measurements of repetitions in the identical text.

(4) Adaptation in stuttering

To complete the balbutiogram it is also necessary to determine the adaptation effect. This is of therapeutic interest because the absence of an adaptation effect suggests the possibility of a cluttering component or also an organic basis, which implies the need for a medical explanation (points 1.7 and 1.8). Measurement of the adaptation effect is similar to that of the consistency effect but here it is the continuing decrease (in contrast to the constancy and even the increase) in the frequency of stuttering as a function of the number of readings of the same text under constantly maintained conditions. Usually, a moderately difficult text of about 100 to 200 words is read five times successively without long pauses.

1.4. Concomitant Symptoms

Observation is extended to those areas of behavior not concerned with speech in a narrow sense but which in the course of symptom development have emerged as accessory conspicuous behaviors. They are usually crucial elements in the symptom complex.

What is meant here are observable concomitant motor movements that occur simultaneously with stuttering (so-called parakinetics). These unconventional and at times very intense movements and tensions of face and neck muscles, of extremities, indeed, even of the entire body need to be described as carefully as possible.

To what extent there is impairment of the capability of the client to express himself or herself nonverbally as by mimicking and by gesture needs to be assessed.

Does the client resort to mimicking and gesture to camouflage or steer clear of symptoms? Are these used somewhat as a bridge across pauses or as nonverbal starters?

Do "reasonable" signs or "inconspicuous" pantomime accompany speech?

The extent or the absence of conventional speech-accompanying gestures should also be noted.

Is body posture tense? Are there alternating periods of tension and relaxation?

To what extent is the client able to establish and maintain eye contact or is this absolutely avoided?

Here, too, as careful consideration as possible should be given to termination of accessory symptoms during several stuttering sequences.

Note: In order to be able to make observations of symptom courses that are as similar as possible to initial collection of data and in subsequent measurement of change it is advisable to standardize sampling of behavior. Thus, the same portion of text can be read by the client at the outset and at various times during the course of therapy. One tape recording can be analyzed with respect to variously formulated questions (for example, features of speech motorics, linguistic and semantic aspects, concomitant movements, etc.).

1.5. Variability in Stuttering

Here the influence of varying conditions on the changeability of stuttering is investigated, especially those conditions that increase or reduce the auditory self-control of speech. Does the stutterer make a deliberate effort to achieve auditory self-control of speech, that is, to produce as fluent speech as possible? How does he or she try to produce actual symptom-free speech? Can he or she describe it verbally?

In cases of such auditory self-control of speech, conditions need to be set up to render it more difficult and eventually to eliminate it.

(1) Whispered reading

Whether the frequency of stuttering in whispered reading of the same text that was read aloud is significantly reduced or not (using a percentage or a statement) needs to be determined. In order to rule out the adaptation effect a suitable time interval (approximately 30 minutes) between repeated readings is reasonable.

(2) Reading and white noise

Reading a text aloud while white noise is presented over earphones to prevent the client from controlling his or her speech acoustically is measured (again, using a percentage or some specification of reduction of stutterings compared with reading of text equally loud under similar conditions without noise).

If a white noise generator is not available auditory self-control of speech can be reduced or curtailed by presenting loud music over earphones.

(3) Rhythmic speaking

A portion of text is read loudly and rhythmically in time with a moderately rapid beat of a metronome (about 80 to 120 beats per minute) (specify reduction in stutterings compared with normal reading). In this situation the attention of the client is diverted from his or her own speech to externally governed control (Chapter 6). A similar effect can be achieved by contriving the following variable conditions:

(4) Simultaneous speaking

Therapist and client read aloud the same text simultaneously in the course of which the client adapts to the reading of the therapist as best as he or she can (slow or fast, loud or soft). The purpose of this is to direct the auditory attention of the client to the speech of the therapist (specify reductions in stutterings compared with reading alone as above).

(5) Varying the situation

Another element affecting conditions under which stuttering occurs involves the social stimuli that may increase or decrease stuttering. At this stage there should be just a compilation of conditions and not a functional interpretation of their interrelations.

Conditions are next recorded that precede stuttering or coincide with its onset, noting how intensely they evoke stuttering (eventually yielding a hierarchy of social situations from negligible to very marked stuttering). The characteristics of the stuttering need to be clarified at least in the following situations:

The client speaks alone.

The client speaks with one and/or several members of his or her family and/or friends.

The client speaks with one and/or several strangers.

The question is: Can the client reveal with which persons or groups of persons in his or her social environment he or she is able to communicate significantly better or significantly worse?

Are there other complicating conditions, such as pressure of time, subject matter, telephone conversations, unfamiliar and increasing complexity of situations, increasing number of listeners, etc.?

With whom and under what conditions does the stutterer not talk at all (avoidance or escape reactions)?

In need of clarification is whether alternative reactions are available to the client in those social situations that are likely to trigger stuttering (for example, written communication or even sign language or shifting responsibility to other persons).

Are there also social situations in which the stutterer speaks fluently without symptoms?

Furthermore, the conditions that ensue from the stuttering need to be sorted out. Here, too, it is important to determine in detail which distinctive aspects of behavior (for example, more or less conspicuous stuttering) lead to what particular consequences (for example, silence or termination of eye contact with an interlocutor; or the turning away from the stutterer, or helplessness and bewilderment of participants in conversation; and also termination of talking in sentences by interlocutors, their sympathy, their amusement, etc.).

1.6. Cognitive Aspects of Stuttering

In this context those cognitive aspects of behavior need to be set out to which problem-determining functions can be provisionally ascribed since they regularly accompany, precede, or follow symptomatic stuttering. Below we follow rather loosely a classification proposed by Fiedler (1978a). Access to cognitive aspects is gained either by engaging in conversation with the client or by direct exploration in which direct communication is required (for example, as organized below). This enables probing of subjective verbal reports.

(1) Stimulus assessments

We are concerned here with the subjective verbal estimation by the client of stimuli and constellations of stimuli. Included are the assessments of social stimuli expressing the extent of their threat or their appeal. (For example, "Fellow workers have little sympathy for my stuttering" or "When I talk with one person he or she listens quite calmly, but with several?!") Whether the assessment of situations is communicated by the stutterer seldom, often, or always in this way should be noted.

(2) Assessment of experiences

Here the cognitive-affective experiences of the stutterer with internal and external stimuli need to be brought together. These are mostly anticipations of continuation or change in emotional state in the presence of actual or expected stimuli (for example, "When the telephone rings it runs ice-cold down my back!" or "When I have to go to the boss my whole body always begins to quiver because I know that once again I won't be able to get out a single word" or "Here in therapy I am always completely calm and relaxed; that's why I hardly stutter"). The extent to which assessments of experience and expectancy fears are correlated should be explored and specified. Expectancy fears reflect the experience that certain situations give rise to increasing autonomic activity and expectancy results in anxieties generated by the respondent himself or herself. Fear of talking should be especially noted (as fear of conversation with particular persons, fear of articulating particular words, etc.).

(3) Assessment of behavior/expectancies of competence

Here we are dealing with the subjective verbal assessments of competency in and capacity for social interaction. They have grown out of experiences in diverse recurring situations. These are evident in various stimulus-generated assessments of behavior (for example, "In the morning it is especially difficult for me to speak without stuttering" or "When I have drunk alcohol I generally speak fluently" or "On the telephone I can't utter a word") and in consequence-dependent assessments of behavior (for example, "When in an interview I really stutter the first time I notice that the interest in me has faded" or "I say nothing in applications about my speech disorder so that I might be first accepted" or "Often I say nothing because no one is listening to me").

(4) Regulation of behavior

Because of their semantic features the subjective verbal aspects of behavior that have been previously set out have a clearly distinctive behavior-regulating (self-generated) quality. In order to work out this aspect even more clearly, it is well here to explicate the regulatory aspect of behavior (allowing the stutterer to do the explicating). This can be done in the form of a behavior regulator list compiled by the client and therapist together.

In so doing it is meaningful to distinguish between stimulus-directed regulation (for example, "When the telephone rings at home I never answer if someone else is in the house" or "I always argue with fellow workers") and consequence-dependent regulation (for example, "I say nothing if my opinion is not sought" or "I frequently say nothing and thus do not attract attention"). Often regulation is due to preceding as well as succeeding stimuli (for example, "When I stutter it is because I have not had my sleep and thus I must have a fear of failure" or "Shopping is difficult for me; I shop mostly at a supermarket so I don't have to ask any questions. I don't shop in a bakery because there I must specify what I want").

Regulatory behaviors that determine the client's latitude of activity are very important. They can be considered further from three points of view:

(a) approach to speech situations
(b) regulating escape from speech situations
(c) regulating avoidance of speech situations

Related to these three points still another subdivision (hierarchy) is possible: (a) regulations that apply rather generally ("metaregulations") and (b) regulations that apply to rather specific situations and behavior consequences.

In accordance with these four points the subjective verbal reports of the client are then simply listed without evaluating whether or not they are factual but, if possible, noting which problem-determining factors can be attributed to them. This will be done in relation to other items under point 4.1.

1.7. Organic Variables

As we stated in Chapter 2 a purely organic cause of stuttering is rather exceptional and, as noted in the propositions contained in our model (Chapter 4), is definitely ruled out as applying to the notion of a continuously developing disorder beginning in early childhood (onset from 2 to 5 years of age). However, organic conditions as associated causal factors need to be thoroughly considered (and this also since early childhood). For this reason medical examination for clarification of any associated somatic causes of the disorder is indicated in every case.

Even if a somatic basis for stuttering is found it does not mean that a psychological-therapeutic factor does not apply to the situation. For, as a consequence of primary organic damage, secondary abnormal behaviors can frequently develop which can usually be influenced favorably by psychological-therapeutic methods. Furthermore, this applies to various manifestations of the speech disorder itself.

All other organic causal factors that have a direct or indirect bearing on the speech disorder can be included under this heading. Prominent in this context are the continuing organic disturbances of function (for example, brain damage, impairment of sense organs, and hormonal difficulties, etc.) (see also point 1.8). Short-term disturbances of function (for example, hyper- or hypoactivity) should be mentioned only if stuttering occurs or fails to appear solely under these conditions or if these conditions clearly alter the probability of occurrence (Schulte, 1974).

1.8. Genesis of Stuttering

The compilation of data concerning the genesis of symptoms concludes this phase of symptom description. They contribute little to a client's "insight" into the development of his or her problems. Rather, genetic analysis provides additional information that contributes to a differential diagnosis and an assessment of factors involved in problems (Schulte, 1974). For this purpose the following areas need to be addressed:

(1) The onset of conspicuous stuttering

When did the stuttering symptoms first occur and attract attention and when were they first diagnosed as "stuttering?"
Who first made the diagnosis of "stuttering?"
As well as it can be determined, what did the marked speech disturbances look or sound like at the onset of stuttering?
Are there earlier diagnostic opinions or therapeutic reports?

(2) Causal factors

To what causes was/is the disorder attributed by the stutterer, the reporting caretaking individuals, and other involved persons such as previous therapists?
Is there a medical assessment of causes? (If not, this should be obtained in every case.)
In this connection the following particular questions need to be addressed:

(a) Can an early childhood brain damage be considered as an associated factor (for example, as in premature birth or forceps delivery)?
(b) Along with the speech disorder can possible cerebral disturbances of movement be involved and also represent a concomitant causal factor of the speech disorder (for example, as with hemiplegia, athetosis, choreoathetosis, chorea)?
(c) Did stuttering follow a skull fracture or brain injury?

(d) Were there traumatic events that might be considered as possible associated causes (for example, war injuries, accidents, experience of fright)?

An affirmative answer to one or more of these questions does not conclusively indicate a related cause, but it does add to a more accurate medical assessment (see also general remarks on point 1.7).

(3) Development of the disorder

Was the severity of stuttering constant or were there continuing deteriorations or improvements?

Are/were periodic fluctuations noticeable (periods of stuttering and not stuttering, spontaneous remissions, etc.)?

Were there significant events in the developmental history of the stutterer following which stuttering was intensified or reduced?

(4) Rearing characteristics

How did caretakers and other related people behave at the onset of the disorder when symptoms actually appeared?

After the determination or diagnosis that the child stuttered what kind of rearing style and manner of behaving did the caretaker adopt?

What changes in rearing behavior were instituted in the course of symptom development?

(5) Hereditary factors

Are/were there other persons who stutter/stuttered (parents/ancestors)?

Are/were these persons close (in a rearing capacity) to the client (pointing to a possible model and imitation learning)?

2. DESCRIPTION OF SOCIAL DIFFICULTIES AND ADDITIONAL CONSPICUOUS BEHAVIORS

Along with speech disturbances we usually find other conspicuous behaviors especially in social contexts, which must also be carefully analyzed. The extent of analysis of social behavior is all the more urgent the longer the disorder has continued and the earlier it had begun.

Additional problem areas in social behavior need next to be identified and organized. This kind of delineation of various problem areas is preliminary and will be discussed again within the framework of analysis of all conditions.

2.1. Specific Conditions

Every individual problem area should be accurately and properly described in the manner suggested by Schulte (1974) and others. However, for orientation the single steps in so doing are set forth briefly:

(1) Description of symptomatic behavior

(a) Topography and intensity differentiated according to motor, subjective-verbal (cognitive), and physiological aspects.

(b) Frequency and oscillation of behavior (referred to some baselines).

(c) Specification of the types of symptoms (forms of inadequacies in social contexts, frequent or infrequent emergence of problems, inability to cope with problematic situations).

(2) Stimulus reactions

Preceding and following stimulus conditions and manner of behavior as well as specification of alternative reactions and notation of effective or ineffective attempts at self-control by the client.

(3) Organic variables

A more detailed description of problems related to various aspects of social behavior is carried out. These are directly related to the social determinants of the problem behavior and they should include the general living conditions of the stutterer.

2.2. Social Analysis

As Innerhofer (1974) has suggested, a social analysis should at least address the following three areas: (a) intimate area (family, spouse); (b) regular activity and work area (school, classes, work groups, colleagues, etc.); and (c) social area (contemporaries, friends, other related persons, etc.). Here it is essential to understand the style and the norms of the milieu to which the client is exposed and the function they serve in determining behavior. Such a social analysis is also extended to other areas (for example, restricted or broad participation in civic affairs or membership in a church), insofar as they constitute normative and behavior-regulating influences.

It will also be necessary for us to return to social analysis within the analysis of all conditions (point 4).

3. DIFFERENTIAL DIAGNOSIS OF THE BOUNDARIES OF THE SPEECH DISORDER

Before preparing a concrete plan of therapy two additional steps are necessary: (1) Should a preliminary decision based on differential diagnosis now be made as to whether the present speech disorder is stuttering or another kind of communication disorder having similar symptoms? (2) In case of a diagnosis of "stuttering" does the present information warrant conclusions about the nature, the cause, and maintenance of the stuttering, that is, does it generate a hypothetical model of the stuttering syndrome that in the subsequent planning of therapy serves as a basis for selection of procedures for therapeutic intervention? We proceed to the differential diagnosis:

On the basis of salient delimiting signs we can determine whether the symptomatology of stuttering is or is not present overall. But here, too, we can make mistakes, especially when there is an overlay of variable patterns of disorder.

3.1. Stuttering and Cluttering

Here we shall limit ourselves to listing a few essential differences between stuttering and cluttering. They are given in Table 5-1 (see also Chapter 1).

Stuttering can occur along with cluttering. We refer to this as stuttering with a cluttering component. If cluttering predominates then cluttering-stuttering exists. Böhme (1977) recommends that treatment be geared to the predominance of either stuttering or cluttering symptomatology. If the reader wishes to go into this subject in greater depth, reference is made especially to Van Riper (1970), Weiss (1950, 1964), Freund (1934, 1952), and Schmidt (1969).

3.2. Stuttering and Stammering

Stammering is characterized by faulty articulation or an inability to articulate specific sounds or combinations of sounds. Usually, the sound is incorrectly spoken or is replaced by another sound. As is the case with stuttering, stammering is also a transitional stage in normal speech development (between ages 2 and 4). However, it is questionable whether it persists beyond age 4. Symptomatic stammering is thought to be caused by abnormalities in areas involved in articulation (anomalies of tongue, teeth, palate) or brain injury. It has also been observed as a consequence of faulty neurotic development and, thus, can be acquired by imitation learning (for example, by an imitation of a stammering contemporary or

Table 5-1 Differences between Stuttering and Cluttering*

Features	Stuttering	Cluttering
rate of speech	frequently slow	mostly rapid
talking with negligible demand for communication responsibility	better	worse
characteristics of speech	presence of clonic or tonic symptoms	"cluttered" repetitions of words and sentence fragments
alertness in stressful situations	impaired	improved
reading aloud a familiar text	better	worse
soft (whispered speech)	better	worse
speaking with delayed acoustic feedback	improved	impaired
fear of particular sounds	exists	absent
consciousness of disturbance	intense	generally absent
gesture	reduced, inhibited	liberal, uninhibited

*Adapted from Weiss, 1967.

caretaker). This is very often noticed in sigmatism, a faulty "lisping" production of the "s" sound. For diagnosis and therapy of stammering, see Westrich (1978), as well as Führing et al. (1976).

3.3. Stuttering and Symptomatic Iteration

Iteration is characterized by compulsive repetitions of syllables, words, sentence fragments, and sentences, just as they are found in stuttering or cluttering symptomatology. However, iterations occur in organic brain illnesses (for example, central illness in the region of the caudate nucleus) that are not to be confused with stuttering. In addition, many schizophrenics incline toward stereotypic repetitions of word fragments, words, and sentences, often with amazing similarity to stuttering symptoms. We also find iterations in logorrhea, an excessive impulsive flow of speech that is sometimes seen in sensory aphasia. In these cases differentiation from stuttering is accomplished largely by careful analysis of accessory symptoms.

In order to achieve a satisfactory differential diagnosis, collaboration of psychologists, speech therapists, and physicians is a fundamental requirement (see point 5.1).

4. ANALYSIS OF CONDITIONS

From the information collected under points 1 and 2 conclusions about the actual determinants of the stuttering can be drawn. To grasp the manifold individual characteristics and conditions of the speech disorder an ordered evaluation of specific determinants of problems is appropriate at this point.

4.1. Determinants of the Speech Disorder

To begin with, an overall ordering and evaluation of factors that point to a neuropsychological cause for stuttering are called for. The following questions can be helpful:

Are there external conditions under which the stutterer speaks with considerably reduced stutterings (point 1.5. (5))?

Do speech disturbances occur less frequently or not at all under conditions of limited auditory self-control of speech (point 1.5.)?

If this is not the case then somatic conditional factors need to be considered; differential clarification (if need be, repeated) is indicated, especially of organic variables (points 1.7. and 1.8.).

In line with the neuropsychological points of the model developed in Chapter 4, it can be determined here that if the stutterer tries to achieve failure-free articulation by means of auditory self-control then intense, conscious efforts to do so are regarded as responsible for the maintenance of the stuttering. Further clarification of a possible neuropsychological cause of stuttering requires investigation of cognitive (i.e., subjective-verbal) aspects of behavior that can lead to subjectively experienced intensified communication responsibility resulting in concentrated effort to achieve symptom-free speech by means of auditory self-control.

Questions:

When and why does the stutterer strive for auditory control of speech and articulation (point 1.5.)?

Are there sounds/combinations of sounds, syllables/combinations of syllables, words, word fragments, sentences, etc., with which the stutterer takes special pains in anticipation of failure (point 1.6.)?

Do the subjective expectancies (related to loci of difficulty) concur with observed behavior (point 1.3.)?

Are there social conditions under which the stutterer takes special pains to articulate precisely (point 1.6.)?

Under these conditions are stuttering reactions increased and/or intensified (point 1.5.)?

Do the subjective expectancies related to quality and also to quantity of stuttering reactions concur with these observed speech efforts and failure rates? To what extent?

These questions should help in clearly working out the degree to which stuttering is influenced by the subjective effort to achieve failure-free articulation in situations of aggravated communication responsibility.

This general aspect can be broken down more precisely to indicate the conditional factors that control the neuropsychological mechanisms involved in the stuttering. Three questions need to be asked:

(1) Respondent control of behavior

Are these aggravations of activity observed before or during the stuttering and as emotional experiences how do they effect the stuttering cognitively?

The next question addresses specific anxiety reactions generated by social stimuli that precede or accompany the stuttering (point 1.2.). If in almost 100% of observations there is more or less marked intensification directly due to one or more specific stimuli, this can point to a particular condition as a cause of respondent anxiety.

Further to be clarified is whether and how the stutterer anticipates and evaluates changes in intensity of activity (assessment of emotional state, appraisal of experiences) (point 1.6.). Evaluation of experiences possibly affects (as expectancy anxieties) intensification of communication responsibility, which in turn leads to reinforcement of autonomic anxieties.

(2) Operant control of behavior

To what extent do the following stimulus conditions control the speech/stuttering and to what extent do external conditions affect the cognitive approach of the stutterer to his or her speech difficulty? Here the question is how speech behavior is controlled by external stimuli:

Are there situations in which the stutterer speaks willingly? Can these social stimuli serve a positive reinforcing function (approach behavior)?

Are there situations in which the stutterer does not talk? Can these social stimuli serve a negative reinforcing function (avoidance behavior)?

Are there conditions in which the stutterer stops talking (for example, under press of increasing autonomic intensification)? Consequently, can these social stimuli be assigned a negative reinforcing function (escape behavior)?

In connection with this, the kinds of instrumental conditioning that are involved (whether of approach, avoidance, or escape) can, on the one hand, be deduced from the preceding and following external conditions:

> If following symptomatic behavior there is no change in stimulus conditions or if a stimulus condition is produced that has been 'signaled' by the preceding stimulus then approach behavior can be assumed. If, contrary to this, symptomatic behavior changes stimulus conditions so that the preceding stimulus situation does *not* occur then the hypothesis is warranted that escape or avoidance behavior is involved. (Schulte, 1974, p. 87)

On the other hand, this also suggests cognitive behavioral components (point 1.6.), especially stimulus assessment that describes subsequent or changing conditions as "satisfying" or "unsatisfying," as "attractive" or "aversive," as "reassuring" or "not reassuring," etc.

Inquiry into subjective verbal control of behavior can yield additional information that indicates aspects of maintenance (approach) or change (escape and avoidance) of stimulus conditions.

(3) Cognitive control of behavior

To what extent does the subjective verbal portion of the stutterer's behavior influence speech/stuttering?

In addition to the cognitive respondent inputs and the operant mechanisms that have been set forth above in (1) and (2), further internal determinants need to be sought that influence speech/stuttering in social contexts independently. In this analysis of cognitive behavior two areas are involved:

(a) The significance of intrapersonal conflicts for maintenance of stuttering: Fundamental to the specification of intrapersonal conflicts are the recorded assessments and controls of behavior.
Questions:
Are there assessments and controls of behavior that are contradictory? Is there ambivalent control of behavior that leads to uncertainty and helplessness in making decisions?

Following difficult-to-resolve conflicts in social situations is there an intensification of physiological excitation and subsequent resulting fear of symptoms?

The following illustrative twofold approach-avoidance conflict can be noted in a general form in many stutterers and can be specified individually.

"When I talk I meet a social requirement (+), but then I stutter (−). When I am silent no one notices that I stutter (+); however, as a silent one I am left out of things (−) and perhaps irritate the others (−)."

In this example, talking, just as not talking, has appealing (positive) as well as threatening (negative) consequences. Similar conflicts, perhaps complicated even more by social determinants, react upon emotional experience and in this way affect the appraisal of speech competence and consequently subjectively experienced responsibility for communication.

With unresolvable intrapersonal conflicts it should be noted further that habituation to the conflict can mitigate against prevention of external and internal conditions that foster maintenance. This situation often results in a continuing state of excitation and stress reactions (so-called *general activation syndrome*, Birbaumer, 1975). Psychosomatic illnesses of stutterers may possibly be due to such continuing conflicts.

(b) The assessment of personal problems and the subjective estimate of their changeability.

To determine this we can fall back on the recorded behavior and competence assessments as well as on metabehavior controls specified by the cognitive approach to the problem (1.6.). Here we must discuss the extent to which marked rigidity or flexibility can be revealed in these cognitive problem areas. We need to assess how the client judges the possibilities of symptom change or improvement. Such judgments influence therapy to a very great degree. Poor motivation and readiness for change (as well as identification of self as a "hopeless case," repeatedly found among stutterers) have considerable consequences for progress in therapy. If there is an unfavorable premature self-prognosis by the client, often occurring during the diagnostic phase, then a motivating discussion is in order to familiarize the client with the extensive diagnostic therapeutic measures (Fiedler, 1974).

To summarize our analysis of the determinants of stuttering to this point, mutual influences on the speech disorder are outlined in Figure 5-1.

4.2. Determinants of Social Disturbance

Conspicuous features of the speech behavior of the stutterer in social situations have been addressed from several fundamental points of view under 4.1. We must now analyze more precisely those additional determinants which up to this point have only been partially or not at all considered. Here, too, a sequential procedure is indicated: respondent,

Figure 5-1 Influences on Fluent or Stuttered Speech

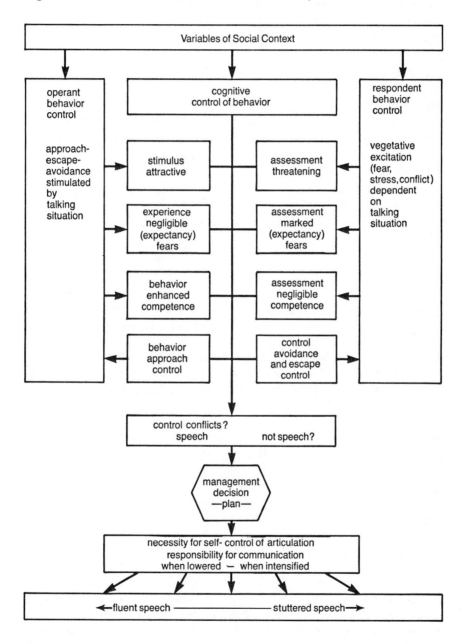

operant, and cognitive conditional factors related to problems of social behavior. Such an analysis can roughly follow the steps given above. In addition, a schema of behavior analysis is helpful (see, for example, Schulte, 1974; Innerhofer, 1974; Fiedler, 1978a).

We shall also call attention to several other points that merit special consideration in analysis of individual speech disturbance.

(1) Social models

We need to determine whether among individuals who interact socially with the stutterer (especially caretakers, parents, teachers, etc.) there are others who likewise had or have a speech disorder (stuttering). This would indicate that models exist for symptomatic behavior (also for typical social behavior). The association of the client with these persons should be understood clearly. We recommend that these individuals be included as much as possible in the diagnosis and therapy and, if necessary, in the therapeutic program itself by participating along with the client in the therapeutic program.

(2) Restricted social activity

The scope of activity of stutterers is considerably circumscribed, especially if symptoms are particularly marked. This is due not only to the clients themselves through internalized views of their problems and social roles, but also to the continuous experience of limiting influence on their activity on the part of those who comprise their social environment. This can present quite a problem for therapeutic efforts to improve social behavior. Therapy directed "against" the environment promises only negligible results. Therefore, analysis of environmental conditions should definitely be involved in planning for therapy. In this context it is pertinent to consider the data collected under point 2 using the following specific headings:

(a) *Intimate and social areas*: What positive or negative consequences for symptoms emerge or have emerged from the designated relationship between close associates (for example, caretakers) and the stutterers? The significance of a change of symptoms for the client and his or her social partner needs to be looked into. It is conceivable that effective therapy would burden close social relations (for example, with a spouse), particularly if the symptoms had served an important function for reciprocal relationships (the spouse may feel responsible for the stuttering—"sick"— partner). Question: When the symptom ceases does the stutterer have adequate social skills at his or her disposal?

(b) *Academic and work areas*: A thoroughgoing investigation of the preschool, school, and occupational circumstances of stutterers is definitely indicated because these can often be the source of severe difficulties. Although academic and occupational skills are hardly, if at all, affected by stuttering, parents and teachers time and again rather emphatically request withdrawal from school when, for instance, stuttering occurs in the first year. Obviously, if symptoms are severe and resist therapy it is absolutely necessary to take school and/or career choice into account. Because of its possible implications for therapy a complete assessment of the individual's occupational skills and interests is in order (for example, through colleagues, in the school psychological service, or by psychological consultation with the employment agency). Furthermore, it is important to know how individuals involved in these occupational areas (teachers, superiors, colleagues) regard the stutterer and his or her symptoms and how they react to them overtly. Is the stuttering tolerated or is it annoying? Is scholastic or occupational advancement made more difficult because of the stuttering? Is the stutterer not required to meet achievement standards and demands because of his or her speech disorder? Over a period of time has this possibly resulted in intellectual and behavioral deficiencies? The answers to these questions will affect the choice of starting points for therapy and the entire therapeutic plan.

4.3. Summary of Analysis

After this detailed analysis of the individual and social conditions of the stuttering it is useful once again to discuss and to assess the relationships among particular areas. At a minimum this should be considered from two points of view:

(1) Development of stuttering and social disturbance

What once again is summarized are when and how the speech disorder took shape and how in the course of symptom development it changed, when and under what circumstances did individual and conspicuous social behaviors come along, and which ones and why were they cultivated? If there are distinctive symptom clusters (for example, stuttering and additional disturbing social behaviors), the extent to which these are related needs to be discussed. Can the origin of symptoms be traced to these relationships (for example, the result of parental rearing attitudes, of traumatic events, of a relapse)?

(2) Direct determinants of stuttering and concomitant conspicuous behaviors

It is important to look into the degree to which varying aspects of symptoms and conditional factors correlate with one another and whether they are reciprocal. Conditions resulting in social anxieties may be due to intrapersonal conflicts as well as to environmental social factors. Intensified responsibility for communication on the part of the stutterer can grow out of actual demands of the interlocutor. This can also happen although the demands of the social situation are not obvious. In the first case symptoms maintained by social conditions while in the second they are mediated by the internally produced cognitions of the client. As much as is practicable therapy should assess the conditions and/or aspects of behavior that call for further consideration of symptom clusters.

5. GENERAL CONSIDERATIONS IN PREPARING THERAPEUTIC MEASURES

Following this analysis a decision needs to be made around what focus therapeutic intervention should be coordinated. A decision of this kind is indeed very difficult if we think of the multivarious conditions, even in the case of an individual stutterer, that are found to be jointly responsible for maintenance of the speech disorder. We shall refer here to several points of view concerning the choice of starting point for therapy. In what follows we shall limit ourselves to a few references, especially since we do not want to deal with specific therapeutic measures. These will be taken up in the next chapter.

5.1. The Need for Interdisciplinary Decisions

The diagnostic task with stutterers requires a closer collaboration of medicine and psychology, much more than with other behavioral disorders. Stuttering may be traced to multiple interrelations between psychogenic and somatic factors. This suggests collaborative search for a therapeutic starting point, the more so if there are additional complex psychosomatic findings combined with stuttering. Symptom clusters and their various actuating and maintaining conditions need to be differentiated. Of course, a differential diagnosis that attempts merely to state whether a causal factor of a symptom cluster is organic or nonorganic is too simplistic. Many more interrelations and correlations among various causal factors need to be worked out to constitute the basis for differential management.

5.2. The Age of the Stutterer

All information about therapeutic potential points to the conviction that early identification and early management of stuttering lead to better prognoses and to optimal therapeutic outcomes (Widlak & Fiedler, 1977; Böhme, 1977). The potential goal of therapy, reduction of subjectively experienced responsibility for communication, is easier to attain in children and youth the less fixed the school or vocational demand for good speech is. The number of caretakers still needs to be considered. Involvement of social partners and educators is almost always imperative and feasible. In the management of children all social interaction should be centrally involved as much as possible. This applies especially to inclusion of parents (as the most important cotherapists). Long-term placement in an institution renders the unconditional necessary contact with parents, siblings, and friends impossible and increases the danger of regression upon return from the institution. Consequently, in cases of children with severely disordered speech, temporary withdrawal from the original social milieu may be necessary in order to achieve initial improvement or to lay the groundwork for therapeutic activity within the social sphere. However, very careful attention must be paid in intramural management to the gradual return of the child to his or her original social setting in order that the speech behavior developed in the institution be carried over into normal life surroundings.

This concludes the synopsis of the diagnostic schema. The supplementary value of psychodiagnostic test procedures is still an open question. In this connection we recommend as worthy of consideration the test procedures of Johnson, Darley, and Spriestersbach (1963), especially "Check List of Stuttering Reactions," "Scale for Rating Severity of Stuttering," "Iowa Scale of Attitude Toward Stuttering," and in any case "Stutterer's Self-Ratings of Reactions to Speech Situations."

The following chapters aim first of all to acquaint the reader with various current interventions in the management of stuttering and to comment on their value and usefulness (Chapters 6 to 9). Then we shall focus on questions of differential treatment of varying symptom pictures and for various age groups (Chapter 10). We shall also refer to our proposed diagnostic schema as we set up goals and decide on choice of methods related to individual findings.

Chapter 6

Management of the Speech Disorder

INTRODUCTION

For almost 2,000 years it was believed that stuttering was due to some difficulty of the tongue. Aristotle (384–322 B.C.) thought that the tongue was too sluggish to keep pace with the ability to conceptualize and communicate. The Roman physician Celsus, who lived at the time of Christ, maintained that it was too frail. Mercurialis (1584) believed that it was too moist and he treated stutterers with a kind of "dehydration therapy." Francis Bacon (1627) applied hot wine to the tongue in order to make it flexible. Demosthenes is said to have resorted to a kind of "self-modification" by loading his tongue with pebbles and thereafter spoke fluently. At the beginning of the nineteenth century this method was again seized upon by Voison, who required the stutterer to take small stones into his mouth. The surgeon Dieffenbach finally achieved morbid notoriety in 1841 for his very painful and frequently fatal operation on the tongue. He transected it at the root or singly removed V-shaped pieces; over 200 individuals were treated in this or similar manner. More of the history of the management of stuttering can be found in Schilling (1965), Van Riper (1973), and Böhme (1977).

Toward the end of the nineteenth century training procedures besides surgical and prosthetic methods were recommended for the first time. In the first half of that century recognition of their results caused such training (and psychotherapeutic) procedures to find their way into the management of stuttering more and more. Increasingly, serious attempts were also made employing combinations of procedures to integrate music therapy, physiotherapy, depth psychology, and finally logopedic and pedagogical approaches (Gutzmann, 1898; Froeschels, 1924; Liebmann, 1914). Still, convincing conclusions could not be drawn despite reporting from time to time of results of differing approaches. Finally, especially in the German-speaking area, an interdisciplinary dialogue had its inception and has been carried on fruitfully to the present time (Schilling, 1965; Böhme, 1977). In recent years these deliberations have been greatly enriched, especially by Anglo-American research (Sheehan, 1970a; Van Riper, 1973).

In the preceding chapters we attempted to make clear that the speech disorder of stuttering is multifaceted, socially as well as neuropsychologically. A complex substratum of internal (neurological and cognitive-emotional) conditions and manifold environmental factors underlies stuttering. In order to do justice to the polyetiology and multisymptomatology of stuttering various methods of treatment are currently combined for the most part with one another and are employed in therapy simultaneously or in rational sequence. Significantly basic to this are psychotherapeutic methods, especially behavior therapy, which is frequently associated with medical, logopedic, and sociopedagogical management.

The increasing effort to integrate a variety of therapeutic techniques has resulted in vast differences in therapeutic programs. Nevertheless, structural similarities are evident when the uses of diverse combinations of management are assessed. Hence, probing for varying focal points of emphasis during the course of therapy takes into account the multivaried nature of stuttering. Areas of intervention can be roughly delineated as follows:

1. Treatment of the speech disorder
2. Preceding and concomitant measures in the treatment of the speech disorder
3. Establishment of self-control of fluent speech
4. Management of social difficulty
5. Combined and overlapping management procedures as well as additional psychotherapeutic measures.

This delineation of potential points of emphasis facilitates more confident specification of a feasible sequence of therapeutic steps. Ultimately, of course, the sequence depends on the individual features of the disorder (thus, on individual origins, time of onset, age of the client, environmental conditions, etc.). We shall return later in more detail to the question of rational coordination of various procedures and to the question of initiation and implementation of individually tailored programs of therapy (Chapter 10). However, in order to approach our presentation of therapy more systematically, in this section we shall orient ourselves to areas of intervention. We shall next present various methods of treatment of speech and social difficulties successively and discuss their effectiveness and practicability.

The procedures presented in this chapter are aimed directly at relief of the speech disorder. They seek to reduce stuttering by speech therapy. Continuous effort needs to be exerted to break down long-standing aberrant (motor) speech patterns and to reconstruct them by fresh training methods.

If we proceed on the assumption that at the basis of stuttering are neuropsychological mechanisms that are influenced essentially by social and cognitive determinants, then it follows that speech training procedures address only a very restricted area of stuttering symptomatology. Isolated and detached from other measures (for example, social therapy), they are hardly promising, and as experience has shown, the range of procedures themselves is very restricted (Chapter 11). We emphasize that the therapeutic techniques presented in what follows make sense only if they are integrated as elements in a framework of comprehensive management.

SYSTEMATIC TRAINING IN NEW SPEECH HABITS

The goal of many methods is systematic training of new ways of talking that are not particularly consistent with stuttering. Conspicuous symptomatic motor patterns in breathing, phonation, and articulation are eliminated (Seeman, 1969; Hartlieb, 1969; Becker, 1970; summarized by Orthmann & Scholz, 1975).

Early forms of management focused primarily on altering breathing behavior during speech and on systematic relaxation of the speech musculature. As far back as 1879, Instructor A. Gutzmann recommended a technique that he called "speaking the vowel," in which he tried to combine both aspects. Along with breathing exercises this technique included (1) softer and deeper vocalizing, (2) starting with an aspirate, (3) prolonging the initial vowel in a sentence, as well as (4) a "vocal" binding of successive words as the whole sentence was "articulated as one word" (p. 11–12). Gutzmann's propositions were further developed by his physician son, H. Gutzmann, Sr. (1898, 1912). Along with breathing and voice exercises which he took from his father, H. Gutzmann recommended articulation drills to lead the stutterer past the stage of mimicking and gesture to normal speech through conscious action of all muscle groups involved in the speech act. The main point in contributing to effectiveness of the procedures was that they be carried out with conscious attentiveness: "When the stutterer is aware: thus and so must I speak, that is the way all other people speak, if I speak according to rule then I *cannot* stutter at all—then the problem of psychological treatment is solved— precisely nothing more is needed" (1912, p. 437). In recommendations for training, twelve rules of speech served as a useful guide (1926, p. 40):

1. Be calm when you speak, you know you can speak very well!
2. Also speak calmly and slowly! (Syllable by syllable, word by word, sentence by sentence.)
3. Before speaking you must reflect! (First think then begin!)
4. Before speaking you must breathe in briefly and deeply through your open mouth!
5. Speak neither too loudly nor softly!
6. Don't be too lazy to speak (taciturn)!
7. (After inhaling) never direct the exhaled stream of air on consonants but always on the vowel!
8. Never press hard in producing a sound!
9. Begin the open vowel softly, gently and in a somewhat deeper voice!
10. Prolong the first vowel in an utterance and connect all words of a sentence with one another as though all of it were one word!
11. Always speak clearly and pleasingly to the ear!
12. Do not pay attention to the movements of speech but listen to the melodiousness of your voice!

H. Gutzmann's recommendations for training were widely accepted. His speech training book (which his son H. Gutzmann, Jr., recently edited) appeared in 23 editions up to 1966. That this approach to treatment was often also discredited is due chiefly to the fact that frequently procedures were too rigidly structured in accord with the system and too infrequently were they tailored to the individual characteristics of the client's disorder. This led to failures, a hazard to which Gutzmann, Jr., clearly referred (1927; Orthmann & Scholz, 1975). Criticism was directed at an array of similar training procedures that had found acceptance around the turn of the century; the best-known among these were those of Wyneken (1868), Coën (1886), and Kussmaul (1910).

Training in new speech habits, particularly as it is practiced by logopedists, is currently carried on in a more extensive context (Böhme, 1977, Hartlieb, 1969; Becker, 1970). The total speech situation is taken into account in every case and an attempt is made to relate it to therapy. Thus, systematic drilling in new ways of talking goes beyond training in phonemes (sound classes that signal meaning), morphemes (word elements carrying the slightest significance with respect to standards of speech), and sentences in which the meaningfulness of communication of corresponding mimicking, gesture, signs, etc., is included. These extensive training procedures are aimed further at completely forcing open internalized communication gestures (possibly acquired over the years) and relaxing tenseness by training in new gestures. That the use of speech gestures as a medium in therapy has had promising results, especially in the treatment of stuttering in children (Chapter 10), has been repeatedly observed (Calavrezo, 1965, and others).

Speech Gestures

As an illustration we have chosen for more specific comment the work of Calavrezo, which we ourselves observed in 1973.

In Calavrezo's opinion the speech of stutterers reveals a far-reaching lack in stress patterns—the melodic (intonation), dynamic (intensity), and temporal (duration) patterns characteristic of normal speech rhythm. In fact, Calavrezo looked upon this as one of the most important gestalt factors of speech, inasmuch as it contributes to the organization of what is being communicated (1965). Furthermore, there is a deficit of appropriate speech-accompanying gestures, which for the most part are replaced by symptomatic accompanying gestures (expedients such as finger snapping and other parakineses). Gestures affect the talker kinesthetically and the person being addressed optically. Finally, these nonverbal forms of expression are important elements in thoroughgoing communication and expression of the talker.

Consciously inserted gestures help in eliciting normal and fluent speech in therapy. As a training text for this purpose a systematic plan for effective nonverbal and verbal forms of expression should be mutually drawn up by therapist and client, word for word and sentence for sentence. The examples should be so chosen that they allow exaggerated, accented mimicking and gesture, a large variety of rhythm and speech patterns.

For example: enumeration of items in a room, enthusiasm, greetings, oaths, calling for a person, requesting action of an interlocutor, etc. Several illustrative sentences that Calavrezo liked to use: "Our opinions bounce off one another" or "He places the book from one side to the other" or "I come to you because I want to see you and would like to lock you in my arms" or "The glider draws broad circles in the sky. It soars high and falls low. It vanishes out of sight far behind the clouds."

Gradually, these sentences are drawn from colloquial speech and are then adapted to the day-to-day speech of the stutterer. Repetitions of fairy tales and exciting stories with children are suitable for transition.

The stutterer must be able to persevere in systematic drilling should the planned regime of speech and gesture be disagreeable. The therapist has an important motivating function, especially in encouraging resolute utilization by the stutterer of unfamiliar articulation, mimicking, and gesture. Speech rhythm in reading can be required of school-age children and adults. Sentences from suitable texts can be segmented into thought units ("The child/reads/in this rhythm"). Speech pauses and intonation are thus controlled precisely.

Calavrezo claims long-lasting results in about 60% of adult clients if daily therapy can be carried out for 5 to 10 weeks. In 1973 we ourselves observed successful results with children who required less than 4 weeks of treatment in every case. An important precondition for the use of this method is the willingness of clients to accept greatly exaggerated speech and gesture activity, which is quite a departure from a normal standard in the beginning of treatment. Here we also observe how stutterers shy away from forceful gesticulation in struggling valiantly to be as inconspicuous as possible.

In considering the neuropsychological hypotheses of our model we propose two kinds of explanation and evaluation. These effects are less likely to take place if in treatment situations we avoid pressure to achieve and compulsion for results in talking and gesturing. Poorer results are to be expected the more the stutterer in trying to improve his or her speech feels bound to control it by ear. We have already referred to this paradox several times. The training procedures that have been mentioned (especially the gesture therapy of Calavrezo) are presumably more promising if one is able to turn the attention of the stutterer away from self-control of articulation to total exploitation of his or her communicative (also nonverbal) competence. It is certainly worthwhile to introduce this kind of training into therapy in order to relax the expressive behavior of the stutterer. By following modeling by the therapist the client can be accustomed and motivated to relaxed speech and can overcome existing inhibitions more easily. We concur in the judgment that Calavrezo is an excellent therapeutic model. We believe that a great deal of the results with his method are accounted for by his personal therapeutic skill.

"Blowing" While Talking

A type of therapy that concentrates on modification of breathing and speech habits of stutterers has been recently described by Schwartz (1977). In Schwartz's blowing technique aimed at preventing tension in the laryngeal region, particularly spasm of the vocal bands (laryngospasm), an inaudible aspirate precedes the speaking of words. This recalls the "breathing" method proposed by A. Gutzmann in 1879 (see above). In this procedure the client begins talking with an "audible" sigh. Gradually this is switched to voiceless "blowing." During the lesson and the initial use of the method the stutterer needs to be careful not to force his or her speech (and with it the "blowing"). This can happen under stressful conditions. To avoid stuttering, speech must be produced very slowly. Interruption of the breath stream (from the blowing) before the actual production of words also results in spasms of the vocal bands and with it stuttering. The aim of blowing is to set the vocal bands into vibration by "gently" emitting a stream of air always before the beginning of a word and then to maintain it in speaking a sentence. This requires very thorough training since habituation to this new breathing and speech behavior appears only after 16 weeks (Schwartz, 1977). In most cases this procedure evidently enables stutterers to achieve immediate and extensive symptom-free speech in therapy.

Schwartz speaks of a cure rate of between 80 and 90%. These claims appear to be very high (Chapter 11) and are not generally acceptable, especially since no control studies involving these procedures have been reported. Schwartz himself qualifies his claims by stating that the blowing technique is functional only if it is consciously and continuously put into action. Failure occurs if stressful and demanding circumstances interrupt stutterers and when they "forget" the conscious applications of the technique. Therefore, an essential element of the therapy involves transfer of the learned aid to demanding social situations. For this purpose caretakers, among others, are included in the therapy (as mentors). Furthermore, Schwartz appoints his patients as "docents" who initiate other stutterers in the developing and changing conditions of the speech disorder and instruct them in the use of the "blowing" technique. Finally, he brings interested stutterers together into groups with common cultural background (see also our implementations for transfer in Chapters 9 and 10).

Operant Procedures

Supplementing both of the preceding sections are studies dealing with the use of operant and instrumental conditioning to expedite the acquisition of new speech habits (see also Chapter 3). According to the operant learning paradigm, consequences that follow a particular kind of behavior determine the future probability of occurrence of that behavior. Manipulation of consequences enables control of adequate or inadequate responses. This has already been put to the test in a large number of behavior disorders involving children and adults (among others, Kuhlen, 1972; Karoly, 1977; Sandler, 1977). In the treatment of stuttering the aim is to achieve an increase in speech fluency and a reduction in stuttering essentially by means of reward (behavior reinforcement), punishment, or some combination of these. Operant procedures are also introduced to build up non-verbal behavior and to eliminate secondary symptoms (for example, parakinesis). We present an overview of relevant work.

Rickard and Mundy (1965) reported on the treatment of a young man by means of behavior reinforcement of fluent speech. At first, satisfactory results were achieved in therapy sessions and in real-life situations through verbal social reinforcement (for example, "good," "very good") and then later through material reinforcement. However, after 16 months these results were not maintained. Russel, Clark, and Van Sommers also worked with reinforcement of symptom-free speech (1968). Although the study was intended as an experiment and not as actual therapy, their clients also showed a decided generalization to everyday situations along with an improvement in speech. Visual and auditory reinforcers of behavior were used along with verbal and nonverbal ones (also called *token systems*; see Ingham & Andrews, 1973b). For this purpose Tunner (1973) used a res-piration feedback device as visual feedback of regular breathing. However, Perkins (1973a) considered the "feeling" of a stutterer that he or she had spoken fluently ("self-reinforcement") to be a far better reinforcer than other operant reinforcing procedures.

Many investigators studied the effect on symptomatic stuttering of administering contingent aversive (punishment) stimuli. Flanagan, Goldia-mond, and Azrin (1964), reporting on three of their clients, stated that they achieved a reduction in the frequency of stuttering by contingent punish-ment of every symptom. As an aversive stimulus an unpleasant 600 Hz tone at 105 dB was presented over earphones for one second. Biggs and Sheehan (1969) got similar results using a 4,000 Hz tone as the average stimulus. Under controlled conditions Flanagan, Goldiamond, and Azrin presented the unpleasant tone continuously; however, it was broken off if a speech failure occurred (about five seconds long). Thus, the client could terminate the aversive situation by stuttering (negative reinforce-ment of "escape behavior"). As a consequence of expectancy this resulted in an increase in stuttering.

The uses of anticipatory aversive stimuli vary very much from study to study. They range all the way from insertion of verbal aversive stimuli such as "wrong" or "stop" to the use of such stimuli as harmless electric shock (Martin & Siegel, 1966; Martin, 1968). Siegel and Martin (1967) offer the qualification that many aversive measures are effective only with individuals who have a high failure rate (contingent disfluency was com-municated over headphones by the word "wrong"). However, the changes that were achieved did not last much beyond the experimental phase.

Another kind of punishment is represented by the "time-out" proce-dure. It, too, is used in varying ways. Usually, the stutterer is required to stop talking for a certain period of time after the onset of each symptom (Browning, 1967; Haroldson, Martin, & Starr, 1963; Adams & Popelka, 1971). As a "time-out" condition in an experiment with children Schulze

(1973) introduced termination of eye contact or of any social contact by a turning away of the head of the listener. Egolf, Shames, and Seltzer (1971) used "time-out" in group therapy. The stutterer could speak only as long as his or her contribution was failure free; at the onset of disfluency he or she had to stop talking and the conversation was continued by another member of the group. Within a treatment period of five weeks the number of failure-free words spoken successively by the ten members of the group increased an average of 33.4 to 583.6 words. In referring to this, Adams and Popelka (1971) pointed out that although generally there were positive results during the treatment phase there definitely were individual differences in the effects.

Apart from the observation that stuttering reactions reduced by the use of aversive stimuli do not persist beyond the experimental phase in most cases, Bloodstein (1969) thought that punishment methods can also lead to an increase in anxiety.

In several experiments reward and punishment procedures were combined. Moore and Ritterman (1973) found equivalent effects both by punishing speech disfluencies and by simultaneous reinforcement of fluent speech. It is doubtful, at any rate, whether reward and punishment are essentially different from each other, especially since the absence of reward is probably punishing and the absence of punishment is rewarding. To the present time the problem of the cognitive operation of reward and punishment has hardly been discussed (Fiedler, 1975). Schulze (1973) was able to reduce stuttering in children considerably by combined reward/punishment procedures and by the introduction of additional measures. Mothers of the children were enlisted as therapeutic aides and implementation of the measures devolved essentially upon them. An effort was made first of all to determine the frequency of stuttering (baseline) and to give the children an understanding of what stuttering is and how it is manifested. Punishment stimuli contingent upon stuttering were firmly administered at daily training sessions. In the main these consisted of termination of contact and turning away of the mother. Added to this later was the withdrawal of material reinforcers (tokens). At the end of a training session the child could exchange the remaining chips for sweets or money. It is doubtful whether these results are precisely replicable since among the children in the study there was a clutterer, for whom the particular method was exceedingly effective. Another kind of application of operant methods was illustrated by Egolf, Shames, and Blind (1971). They used reward and punishment to change the attitude toward both stuttering and the person herself.

Shames and Egolf (1976) presented an extensive program for management of adults, adolescents, and children based on systematic application of operant procedures. It entailed detailed recommendations for the use of multiple reinforcement programs aimed at changes in conspicuous behavior as well as modification of speech behavior. The involvement of caretakers who were instructed in operant methods was a prominent component in the therapy.

In general, reports indicate that in most cases reward and punishment procedures are effective only over the short term (exception: Shames & Egolf, 1976). Flanagan, Goldiamond, and Azrin (1964) reported quite a "compensatory increase in stuttering" at the termination of the experimental phase. The neuropsychological hypotheses of the model (Chapter 4) can explain this. During the experimental phase the attention of the stutterer is very intensely oriented to external stimuli (the conditions of reward and punishment). Following the experimental procedure the stutterer concentrates all the more on his or her own speech since the experimental conditions were expected to result in improvement. This kind of auditory self-control of speech leads to an intensification of integration and coordination difficulties, which then precipitate the "compensatory" increase in stuttering.

From this point of view, attention to speech production (fluent or disfluent), rewarding, punishing, etc., is usually not recommended. Rather, the proper effective application of operant methods to improve nonverbal behavior (mimicking gesture, sign language) as well as to eliminate concomitant symptoms is definitely indicated. This needs to be combined with other possibilities for speech management. We shall deal with this further.

Negative Practice

The intervention strategies that have been presented to this point have had as their aim the reduction of symptoms by training in new speech habits. It is implicitly assumed that habituation to normal communication situations would be generalized. We now refer to additional procedures involving negative practice, about which an extensive number of controlled studies have been done (summarized by Widlak, 1977).The idea of therapy based on negative practice (also less frequently referred to as "negative training") was advanced by Dunlap (1942). It was recommended for a wide array of behavior disorders, for example, such as tics, compulsiveness, and also for stuttering. In its therapeutic application the stutterer had to repeat stutterings several times voluntarily and accurately. The exact imitation (mimicry) indicated the characteristics of the speech associated with failure. Negative practice differs crucially from procedures cited previously in that it requires neither control of symptom-free speech nor the avoidance of failure. On the contrary, drilling is on failure, not on failure-free speech.

This procedure is usually theoretically accounted for by the concept of "conditioned inhibition" of Hull (1943; Kendrick, 1960; Kehrer & Stegat, 1968; Manns, 1969). In the course of training, an increasingly strong and growing central inhibitory reaction takes place against the applied procedure by which stuttering inhibits itself; stuttering *can* no longer occur. Fluent speech replaces stuttering, which, so the theory goes, is reinforced by fluent transition to word sequences immediately because it is associated with the comfortable feeling of tension reduction. This behavior is reinforced by frequent repetition.

For practical implementation several specific regimes are proposed (also Lehner, 1960): Two sessions per week (more, if necessary) are held with the client. The first five contacts in therapy normally last about 30 minutes each. Later sessions lasting up to an hour are practicable. About every ten or fifteen minutes an unconditional recess is inserted, since negative practice demands extraordinary client exertion. At any rate the training sessions should extend only over that interval of time during which the client can make progress in his or her effort to foster involuntary reactions by voluntary endeavor.

At first it seems paradoxical to a layman that symptomatic behavior is abolished while practicing it. It is therefore very important to explain repeatedly the purpose and procedures of negative practice in the first session. The client must be prepared to enter into the training since it is very exhausting and enervating.

If, during training, symptoms occur in free conversation or in reading a text, the client is immediately interrupted and asked to repeat the stutterings, including accessory gestures as accurately as possible. In this connection Lehner (1960) refers to the difficulties caused by the stutterer by his or her perception of symptoms and of identical reproduction. But the latter is necessary. The stutterer should *not* practice any procedures for stuttering (nor do it somewhat involuntarily) but should try, indeed voluntarily, to reproduce the form of his or her involuntary stuttering as accurately as possible. Otherwise, there is the danger that merely a new habit has been added to the existing stuttering. That is why Lehner does not advise independent drilling and application of negative practice by clients without the therapist, even by those clients who are making good progress.

As to results (reported among others by Brutten and Shoemaker, 1967; Kehrer and Stegat, 1968; Widlak, 1977), therapeutic failures limit the value of this method. From the statistics of results cited by Lehner (1960) as well as by outcomes reported by Case (1960), it is clear that for tonic forms of stuttering negative practice does not work at all or at least to any satisfactory degree. Worsening of symptoms has also been reported. Furthermore, according to Manns (1969), an increase in stuttering must be reckoned with at the beginning. This is certainly not without its problems, even with clients who are highly motivated for therapy.

It is difficult to state the implications of negative practice for our model (Chapter 4), especially since authors do not often communicate significant background conditions. For example, in assessing successful results of this method should we not seek to determine whether the negative practice was carried out as a kind of achievement-oriented training with the implicit attainable goal of speaking normally in the shortest possible time?

For example, making modest demands on client and caretaker following therapy renders immediate desirable results difficult to attain. We shall return to this point in more detail later (Chapters 10 and 11). Suffice it to say here that negative practice, if used at all, should be included in broadly designed therapy only in conjunction with other procedures.

It is worth noting that negative practice reminds us of the procedures of "paradoxical intention" of the Viennese psychiatrist Frankl (1960). According to this approach, the fear of stuttering is diminished if the client trades his or her presymptom anxiety for the paradoxical intent at this stage to stutter more than ever.

Shadow Speech

In shadow speech the stutterer repeats with slight delay material from a text invisible to him or her that has been read aloud by the therapist (or some other person). During the shadowing procedure the frequency of stuttering is often considerably reduced.

Explanation of this method may be based on the ideas of Cherry and Sayers (1956; also Chapter 2). They advance the hypothesis that stuttering is caused by a defect of perceptive awareness and that by this kind of aid to speech the attention of the stutterer is diverted from his or her own speech to that of the person doing the talking. Such an explanation agrees fundamentally with the ideas of our model (Chapter 4). Shadow speech is controlled externally; auditory self-control of speech is reduced.

It is advisable in therapy to begin with short, slowly spoken sentences that must be shadowed easily by the client. The level of difficulty is gradually increased in that the sentences get longer and the tempo of speech is changed. Cherry and Sayers suggest that sustained training of speech by this method fosters the development of normal feedback control. Their reports of results using these procedures are encouraging. Effectiveness is evidently improved by deliberately introducing difficulties. This is done by having the talker change the tempo of loudness of his or her speech (MacLaren, 1960). Walton and Black (1960) introduced shadow speech among other procedures rather effectively in the case of a client who had marked difficulty in talking over the telephone but whose symptoms were otherwise only mild. Similar improvements in speech using a specified shadowing procedure can be realized when the stutterer tries to follow a tape recorder or speech from a radio (Yates, 1963b). These open possibilities for practice between therapy sessions.

Simultaneous speaking involves the procedure in which the stutterer talks along with another person, such as the therapist, in reading from a text in similar fashion. Here, too, we may anticipate significant symptom reduction followed by symptom elimination. But in simultaneous reading or speaking, the first word of a sentence that the stutterer must give without hesitation frequently poses problems. An interesting additional finding is that the stutterer continues talking with normal fluency on his or her own if after a certain time the simultaneous talker switches to another text while the stutterer continues to read the original text (Cherry & Sayers, 1956).

Simultaneous and shadow speaking recall one of the older methods influencing stuttering, that of Liebmann in 1914, which has been mentioned previously. In the procedures of this unisono-method, simultaneous speaking and reproduction of another talker's speech play a central role (also Schilling, 1965; Orthmann & Scholz, 1975; Böhme, 1977). Recently these procedures have been taken up in the speech laboratory (Blankenheim, 1973). Stuttering children read a text together with the speech teacher. The pupils hear the combined speech over earphones. Then the loudness of the teacher's voice is gradually reduced until the pupil finally speaks by himself or herself. Sentence-by-sentence reproduction of short stories leads to free telling of a story afterwards. Finally, there is practice in free conversation. Blankenheim suggests additional possibilities for the treatment of stuttering in the laboratory.

Aids to speech such as shadowing take on an important helping function in the context of stuttering therapy. However, various authors are rather pessimistic about producing a complete elimination of symptoms or long-standing improvement solely by the shadowing approach. Meyer and Mair (1963) and Ingham and Andrews (1973a) are among the critics. Speech aids, however, which while in use may lead to conditional failure reduction, are generally only a step, although an important one. For example, they may restore to the stutterer once again the feeling that his or her speech disorder is not entirely hopeless. This, above all, is an essential precondition for continuing often wearisome work in therapy.

Masking of Speech Output

By masking is meant the controlled presentation of noise (white noise) over earphones (Chapter 2). This can prevent the auditory control of speech. According to the theoretical views of Cherry and Sayers (1956; Chapter 2), the effect of masking is primarily due to a possible complete switching off of the auditory feedback, including that by bone conduction, especially of the low-frequency portion of the feedback.

A therapeutic approach using this method would seek to produce normal speech under conditions of white noise masking and to establish the foundation for a new motor set for fluent speech. The effectiveness of this method, that is, the attainment of fluent speech under conditions of white noise, appears to depend on the intensity of the masking sound and on the frequency of presentation (Burke, 1969). Maraist and Hutton (1957) obtained a significant clinical effect by using a white noise of 50 dB. They first obtained approximately normal speech by presentation of a mixed frequency sound at 90 dB. But this required level was close to the threshold of pain (Yates, 1963b). This is presumably why high-level masking is rarely included in therapy. Another reason may be that a long-time effect is very difficult to achieve. The majority of these studies were concerned with short-term effects in an observation time frame of about 10 minutes (May & Hackwood, 1966; Adams & Moore, 1972). However, Fineberg-Garber and Martin (1974) obtained longer-lasting masking effects. Sutton and Chase (1961) were able to show that continuous white noise not only reduced the frequency of failure but showed effects for presentation in speech intervals similar to those produced when the given masking noise was presented during speech only. Webster and Dorman (1970) were able to confirm these findings. (See the theoretical considerations mentioned in Chapter 2.) In general, it seems to us that therapy can include both gradual reduction in intensity and intermittently introduced practice.

Reports on suitable masking devices also vary (Perkins & Curlee, 1969; Trotter & Lesch, 1967; Parker & Christopherson, 1963; Van Riper, 1973). Experience suggests that expensive units be purchased only conditionally (or that they be constructed). In their overview Ingham and Andrews (1973a) concluded that masking could result either in improvement or complete elimination of symptoms. Further research is required to evaluate its clinical usefulness for all kinds and severity of disturbance.

Delayed Auditory Feedback (DAF)

In addition to shadowing and masking, there are other measures that lead more or less to reduction and elimination of auditory control of the stutterer's speech and eventually to its fluency. One of these possibilities is delayed auditory feedback (DAF) of the stutterer's own speech (see also Chapter 2). In this procedure the talker's own words are fed back to him or her over earphones with a given time delay, much like an echo. As mentioned in Chapter 2, DAF causes a speech disturbance (especially repetitions) in normal-talking persons resembling stuttering. But in stutterers this results in substantial reduction in hesitations and failures (tonic as well as clonic symptoms). Relatively short time delays (50 to 100 milliseconds) produce significant reductions in failures. Physical behavioral impairments are also reduced (Lotzmann, 1961). The effectiveness of delayed speech feedback in reducing speech hesitations points up its usefulness as a therapeutic tool. Under conditions of DAF, normal-talking persons as well as stutterers consciously try to reduce the disturbing influence of the fed back signal by prolonging speech segments. In so doing they slow down the tempo of the speech.

Various approaches to treatment have taken advantage of this effect. To begin with a strong acoustic signal with a time delay of 200 to 500 milliseconds is used. The client learns to speak as slowly and in as prolonged a fashion as possible. Then the time delay is reduced further until the largest effect on symptom reduction is observed. At this point the stutterer is required (as he or she has previously learned) to maintain the slow and prolonged speech as much as possible. Tunner and Florin (1969) recommend reinforcing the slower speech by additional acoustic or optical stimuli in order to demonstrate to the client his or her progress in therapy. The time delays are successively reduced in the course of therapy (thus approaching the natural acoustic feedback time) until the newly learned manner of speaking can be maintained without technical help. The prolonged manner of speaking developed through DAF is not to be identified with normal speech. However, it is effective in the course of continuing therapy (Goldiamond, 1965; Perkins, 1973a, b). We shall return again in Chapter 10 to the place of DAF as an aid in speech therapy in the context of combined therapy.

Unfortunately, not every therapist has access to a DAF device. Perkins (1973b) and Curlee and Perkins (1973) claimed, nevertheless, that it was possible to obtain the same or similar effects by requiring (and training) the stutterer to speak slowly and in a prolonged manner (so-called *prolonged speech*). This has been tried in a wide array of therapies (among others, Van Riper, 1958, 1973; Schwartz, 1977; and also in earlier speech therapies such as those of Gutzmann, 1926, Coën, 1886, as well as of Wyneken in 1868). An unquestionable advantage of the DAF device is that the rate of speech can be controlled, making possible a methodical approach to normal speech tempo. The "forced" slowing down in manner of speaking also simultaneously stimulates new coordination of breathing and articulation.

It has been found that the effect of DAF differs between men and women stutterers (Van Riper, 1971). There are individual differences in the most desirable delay time for maximum symptom reduction. It should be noted that additional speech failures (notably repetitions) may turn up which are also typical for normal talkers under DAF (negative Lee Effect; Lotzmann, 1961). These need to be overcome by insistent slow and prolonged speech as in the case of normal talkers.

Although relatively symptom-free speech under DAF can be achieved by prolonged speech, therapeutic effects usually do not persist if no additional measures are taken subsequently. These are necessary because the prolonged speech practiced under DAF was unnatural. Moreover, it has been noted that with children DAF can give rise to intense affective-associated symptoms and anxieties (see Chapter 2); therefore, it should not be used with young persons.

Rhythmic Speaking

Efforts to apply speech rhythm as therapy for stuttering have a long tradition. Thus, as far back as 1868 Wyneken, who, as was the case with many authors cited in this book, was himself a stutterer, recommended that the stutterer must "keep time." He recommended that "every sentence as well as multisyllable words be spoken quite slowly, all syllables of the same length . . . and always, just as we insert marks in writing, to indicate when to take a breath" (p. 4).

Since without exception stutterers can speak relatively rapidly and almost symptom free in following a rhythm, it is understandable that therapists of diverse theoretical orientation have investigated the relation of the phenomenon to therapy (Johnson & Rosen, 1937; Barber, 1940; Van Dantzig, 1940; Fransella & Beech, 1965; Beech & Fransella, 1971; Andrews & Harris, 1964; Brandon & Harris, 1967; Van Riper, 1973). Also in many current forms of behavior therapy for stuttering, alteration in speech rhythm is attained by guiding the client to rhythmic speech. This is accomplished in the production of syllables, words, or sentence fragments by presentation of acoustic, tactile, or visual stimuli; however, the latter have been the least suitable.

There are various ways in which stimuli that control speech production can be presented:

1. By a table metronome, conventionally used by musicians to control tempo and time.

2. By a haptometronome. This is a small haptic (tactile) stimulus source specially developed for the treatment of stuttering that can be carried relatively inconspicuously. It puts out gentle mechanical shocks to the finger tips (or to other regions of the hand or forearm). As with the table metronome, the frequency of this tactile stimulus can be varied (descriptions can be found in Tunner and Bruckmoser, 1969; Tunner, 1973; Azrin, Jones, and Flye, 1968).

3. By an electric miniature metronome, also called a pacemaster or micronome. It can be worn behind the ear like a hearing aid. This relatively expensive device allows for separate regulation of frequency of time and intensity. Investigations involving the miniature metronome have been discussed, among others, by Meyer and Mair (1963), Brady (1971), and Berman and Brady (1973).

To elaborate the possibilities for therapeutic use of the metronome we have selected as an illustration the thoroughly detailed procedure presented by Brady (1971), so-called "metronome-conditioned-speech retraining."

At the beginning of therapy the clients receive an overview of the course of treatment; among other things, they are told that

- paced speech is only a preparatory and transitional step to extensive symptom-free speech
- metronome-controlled speech retraining would quickly be adapted to normal speech rhythm
- progressive training under conventional environment conditions is essential in order to ensure generalization of behavior learned in therapy sessions

There are additional preparatory steps to be taken. The metronome rate most suitable for the stutterer needs to be determined. This depends on the severity of the disturbance. For very severe stutterers Brady suggests a frequency of about 40 beats per minute. For moderate stutterers the starting rate can be increased to 80 beats per minute. In every case the stutterer paced by the metronome speaks a simple text without effort (a syllable per beat or, for moderate stuttering, a word per beat).

The goal of the next therapy sessions (as effortless and failure-free speech is attained) is to approximate the rate and cadence of a normal manner of speaking gradually. As a first step the frequency of beats is progressively increased. In training, as with other measures, extensive effortless speech as failure free as possible should be the dominant criterion for the effectiveness of therapy. From the beginning and parallel to the reading from a text it is advisable to take into account assorted difficulties in free talking, for example, using picture description, retelling of stories, and conversation with the therapist during training sessions. In this way the client's fear of talking can be gradually reduced (see also Chapter 9). Between weekly sessions the stutterer has to continue daily practice for 30 to 45 minutes at home similar to that of beginning therapy conducted in formal sessions. If this turns out well, home practice can be carried on in the presence of a person in whom the client has confidence.

In the course of therapy more and more training should be aimed at "normalization" of speech, that is, the elimination of the paced speech. For example, the stutterer should try to say more than one syllable per beat. If necessary the beat frequency may be reduced and then increased again. Transition to words, to short sentences, or to sentence fragments paced by the metronome should be specifically planned. After this the stutterer can use several beats of the metronome for pauses or later vary the number of syllables spoken per beat. In this latter procedure especially, approximation of paced to normal speech is very important. The goal of this phase of the treatment is considered to be achieved if the stutterer can with metronomic support produce 100 to 160 syllables or short words per minute without noticeable blocking. The disfluency rate should not exceed 20% of the rate of the beginning of therapy. In this phase daily home exercises can be carried on in the presence of others.

In a later phase of therapy the table metronome is replaced by a miniature metronome (and also, if available, a haptometronome). The change from one kind of metronome to another may produce regressions. Adjustment in the treatment program is usually made by temporarily reverting to an earlier phase (repetition of preceding training steps). With adaptation to the wearable metronomic device generalization of the learned improvement to the natural social environment of the client begins. To this end a hierarchy of increasingly difficult speech situations is constructed (see also Chapter 9) that lead stepwise to everyday situations. Often in "working through" such a hierarchy unexpected difficulties crop up, especially when the pace continually predominates speech. This can cause the client to avoid social situations again because paced speech, even if it is failure free, is still not a suitable form of communication. In such cases a corresponding speech situation needs to be reproduced in the therapy until metronome-controlled speech is attained that also minimizes the subjective demand on the stutterer for fluency. Here, the inclusion of an interlocutor is a helpful intermediate step (Chapter 9).

The objective of this phase of the therapy is considered to be achieved if the client can really talk fluently and relaxed in all speech situations.

Brady proceeds under the assumption that the metronome beat can serve as a conditioning stimulus for a relaxed state and for anticipation of fluent speech. Thus, the beat of the metronome not only gives the discriminative order "Speak out the next syllable (and the following ones)" but after a certain period of failure-diminished speech it leads to a relaxed attitude toward diverse socially demanding situations.

Finally, the use of the metronome is gradually faded out. This begins in speech situations presenting slight difficulty. Demands are intensified step by step. Here, too, regressions are observed. After a long period of accommodation to the metronome stutterers feel helpless and alone without it. Original fears of talking frequently recur. Stuttering may return with full fury. In such cases Brady advises his clients to orient their speech to an "imagined" internally situated metronome. This can be worked on in therapy. In treating two stutterers Herscovitch and LeBow (1973) succeeded in methodically building up the "imaginary" metronome.

Many clients express the desire to use a micronome or haptometronome permanently or for a long period of time. We comply with this if the client anticipates assistance from it. Brady also sees an advantage in this. He suggests that metronomic support can help the severe stutterer in certain communication situations where he or she is likely to founder without it. The pacer serves for the stutterer a function similar to that of the hearing aid for the hearing-impaired or glasses for the nearsighted.

Necessity for follow-up stems from the experience that time and again regressions occur (see especially Chapter 11). However, these can be cushioned fairly early by reintroduction of a speech aid.

The results reported by Brady using the program described above are encouraging. Of 26 stutterers between the ages of 12 and 53, a total of 23 completed the program. Twenty-one of the clients demonstrated marked improvement both in speech and in general social behavior. Speech records of performance and various questionnaires and interviews were employed to monitor therapy. Monthly follow-up was from 6 months to 3 years.

If metronomic training does not produce desired effects then additional supplementary or alternative methods of behavior therapy can be instituted. Brady mentions, for example, systematic desensitization, delayed auditory feedback, reinforcement of fluent utterances, and, if necessary, cognitive reconstruction. The latter may be indicated if the stutterers yield to the feeling that they are utterly powerless in confrontation with their disorder (see Chapter 8). Negative practice as a supplementary procedure would be inopportune for this. It would weaken the assurance of the client that assisted by paced speech he or she could communicate better.

Modifications of these procedures are possible and absolutely necessary if the individual needs of a variety of clients are to be met. Termination of the program of individual clients may be shaped quite differently to achieve earlier generalizing effects (for example, by early or previously arranged social training; Chapter 10). Nevertheless, in metronomic training it is always helpful to raise the beat frequency slowly and progressively and to construct a hierarchy of speech situations of increasing difficulty to enable the client to confront difficult situations as soon as easier ones have been mastered (Berman & Brady, 1973).

The effect of rhythmic speech is explained for the most part by the discriminative operation of external stimuli on the articulation of syllables and words. A new manner of speaking guided by external stimuli can be developed and maintained. Here, too, our model affords an additional explanation (see also Chapter 4). The attention of the stutterer is diverted from auditory self-control of speech to the pacing stimulus of the metronome. The disturbing influence of the variety of signals fed back by the stutterer's own voice is gone. Pacing of speech by the metronome obviously plays an important part in overcoming auditory awareness. Thus, Tunner (1973) obtained better results using acoustic stimuli as contrasted with tactile ones. Trotter and Silverman (1974) supported this proposition. They observed that the effectiveness of a micronome wore off only slightly after use for a month.

At the beginning of therapy a table metronome has the advantage of enabling the therapist to check easily how and whether the client is maintaining the pace. However, the miniature metronome can be used relatively inconspicuously outside of therapy sessions and, hence, can be helpful in the quest for generalization. Yet, it should be kept in mind that symptom reduction achieved under self-pacing conditions is not inevitably permanent. Tunner presents several examples (1973). In those cases in which the contribution of ''self-reinforcement'' is obviously not sufficient by itself, he recommends the introduction of new or generalized reinforcers in order to improve speech performance once again. In some of his clients fluent paced speech was maintained by changing, among others, the stimulus conditions (replacing an acoustic with a tactile stimulus source). Possibilities for enhancing the efficiency of metronome effectiveness have also been discussed by Brady and Brady (1972) and by Brady (1973). The focus is on a procedure the authors call ''metronome-conditioned-relaxation.''

A number of clients were informed about the relaxing effect of metronome rhythm. The presumption was that this would suggest increased speech fluency. The therapist can take advantage of this effect through additional training in relaxation (see also the next chapter). In metronome-conditioned-relaxation the client is instructed (by Brady in slightly changed form) in the technique of "progressive muscle relaxation" (after Jacobson, 1938). Then brief relaxing instructions are given—for example, "re-lax— re-lax--"—synchronized with the acoustic stimulus at a metronome frequency of 60 beats per minute (or with every second beat at a frequency of about 120 beats per minute) whereby pauses in instruction make sense. In the German language the word *Ru-he* (relax) can be used for instruction. It is anticipated that the coincidence of the metronome rhythm with that of the conditioned stimulus will achieve relaxation or at least reduce tension. This procedure was first successfully used by the authors on an admittedly rather small random sample. It appears to merit further investigation.

The unnatural manner of speech associated with paced stimulation frequently argues against the use of stimulators. It certainly is a disadvantage that a great many training sessions are required to progress from the artificial manner of paced speaking to a normal speech tempo. For this reason stutterers often express an aversion to the procedure and perceive it at times to be just as conspicuous as stuttering itself, even when an aid such as a haptometronome or micronome can be placed quite inconspicuously. This suggests that the method should be reserved only for the severest stuttering configurations. It would be profitable to explore together with the client possibilities for increasing the naturalness of speech even under a pacing regime. Jones and Azrin undertook investigations along these lines (1969). Brady claims that this vouches for the achievement of naturalness of speech following the careful application of his sequence of proposed steps (1971). One can agree with this or not. At the very least it certainly encourages attempts to get closer to the designated goal (see also somewhat similar considerations concerning rhythmic-signal synchronized speech advanced by Mückenhoff, 1976). Finally, it is obviously easier to influence the artificial manner of speaking than the stuttering. The authors mentioned above similarly report that in investigating aids to speech they must also seek a way to proceed from artificial forms of communication to the direct approach to therapy.

FUNDAMENTAL ALTERATION OF SPEECH HABITS

Therapists encounter many and diverse conspicuous behaviors that have previously been fixed in the client's repertoire of behaviors along with the stuttering. This is especially the case with adults. Many years of uninterrupted stuttering undoubtedly lead to a great number of obvious as well as inconspicuous habits, which makes it difficult for the therapist to decide on a favorable point of departure for therapy. In concluding our discussion of the treatment of the speech disorder associated with stuttering we shall consider a procedure that aims particularly to take into account the complexity of stuttering symptomatology. This involves the so-called "short therapy" for stuttering introduced by Azrin and Nunn (1974). Their procedure focuses on the client's ingrained speech habits, which are overcome in a few sessions by the acquisition of a completely new pattern of speech. But there also, additional deviant behaviors need, at least, to be taken into account. Our discussion of this procedure is a logical and proper transition to the chapters that follow.

Azrin and Nunn regard stuttering as a "nervous habit" that they attempt to alter quickly and fundamentally in therapy. They have previously reported results of similar approaches (so-called "habit reversals") to nail biting, thumb sucking, compulsive hair pulling, and other conspicuous behaviors (1973). Based on a variety of investigations they extended the method to treatment of stuttering. The stated aim was to develop a procedure that should accomplish the abolition of stuttering in all everyday situations. It should produce a prompt and enduring result in a minimum of therapeutic time.

Their program is divided into the following progressive segments:

1. First the stutterer is urged to review retrospectively (cognitively and verbally) the development of his or her stuttering. In therapy he or she recalls and verbalizes the unpleasantnesses caused by stuttering up to that time. This kind of initiation of therapy should strengthen the motivation of the client to carry out therapeutic measures. The client is then asked to describe his or her stuttering reactions including concomitant symptoms as precisely as possible. This should also include instances that trigger stuttering such as which words cause special difficulties or what situations or contact with what persons are conducive to stuttering. By this process the stutterer comes to know that his or her stuttering depends on a variety of conditions for which he or she will be better prepared in the future.

   Comprehensive symptom-awareness is extended to include the client's cognitive perception of "anticipations" of stuttering. By a previously arranged signal the client enables the therapist (and conversely the therapist the client) to know when he or she fears the onset of a symptom.

   Based on the assumption that stuttering is generally bound up with a state of heightened tension the stutterer is instructed in techniques of relaxation. In the view of the authors this does not have to happen completely. But the client should achieve the body relaxation as soon as possible, either standing or sitting, that enables him or her to breathe deeply, slowly, and regularly. The self-instruction "relax" ("I am completely calm and relaxed") should facilitate relief from tension.

2. Speech training

The chief objective in speech therapy is to establish patterns of behavior incompatible for the stutterer. If a symptom occurs the client needs to

- stop talking immediately
- exhale deeply and then inhale slowly, thereby
- consciously relaxing the upper part of the body and muscles of the neck ("I am completely calm and relaxed"); then
- consciously formulate a word to be spoken; finally
- speak immediately after inhalation;
- speak the first syllable and words of the sentence emphatically; and
- speak only for a short time (which is extended in succeeding training sessions).

Furthermore, it is important in drilling, that behavior patterns incompatible for stuttering are also carried out in expectation of stuttering. In this way symptomatic behavior can be forestalled. Responsibility for helping, based probably on the findings of the behavior diagnosis (see Chapter 5), devolves on the therapist.

3. Training for generalization

In a next step the client consciously envisages a situation that is difficult for him or her and performs the behavior that has been practiced while thoughtfully trying to go along with the unpleasant situation (similar to *in-sensu* desensitization; Wengle, 1974). The emergency is rehearsed, as it were, in the presence of the therapist.

Then the new breathing pattern is practiced in reading. The number of speech units spoken between breaths is slowly increased. At first the client pauses after each word and, instructed to relax, takes a breath. This is done after every second word, etc. He or she concentrates on this breathing pattern supported by the therapist. Stutterers for whom certain sounds and words require a great deal of effort are stopped and have to repeat them deliberately at various places in sentences.

4. Home assignments

Activities subsequent to the described training sessions are carefully laid out by the therapist. The client is urged to call upon intimate individuals to put up with these new efforts to improve his or her speech and even to have them call attention to the new pattern of talking should he or she forget to apply it. This same circle of persons should make its positive influence felt in achieving improved speech. The stutterer should consciously seek out situations that had previously been avoided and use his or her new manner of talking therein.

It is important to emphasize that the demands made on the time of the therapist are rather modest. Azrin and Nunn report that a single two-hour therapeutic session is usually required from time to time, in which the client receives an entire regime of procedures and these are drilled on. Such single sessions are generally arranged only after several telephone communications. During the first week the therapist carries on three telephone conversations with the client, following which there are longer intervals of time between conversations. From time to time the therapist encourages the client by telephone to use the new pattern of talking and answers questions that may arise.

Azrin and Nunn used these methods with 14 stutterers ranging from 4 to 67 years of age. With the exception of the children, all had previously gone through unsuccessful therapies. Eight clients were symptom free following instruction by the authors. The others achieved symptom reduction of about 80% in the course of which an average diminution in the frequency of stuttering of 94% was already observed one day after the therapeutic session. Data are also presented for individual clients covering a longer period of time. According to the reports of the clients and members of their families, the frequency of participation in conversation with the client increased significantly. Simultaneously, avoidance behaviors associated with individuals and situations that previously evoked stuttering were diminished.

The outcomes that have been achieved by these procedures and the minimal time course involved are amazing, especially since the treatment of stutterers generally requires a great deal of time and yields relatively negligible results (Chapter 11). However, the care with which the above-mentioned investigation was carried out has given rise to some criticism and a good deal of unequivocal skepticism has been expressed about the results. For example, precise descriptions of the individual characteristics and manifestations of the disorder are lacking; ratings and measures of results are based on self-appraisals by the clients. Postmeasurements based merely on frequency counts by the therapist during telephone conversations are presented as objective data. Furthermore, precise descriptions of the behavior of the therapist during therapy sessions are also lacking. The extent to which related persons actually supported therapeutic efforts, as intended, is not ascertainable. The question remains as to whether and to what extent constellations of overall circumstances possibly contributed more significantly to the outcomes of therapy than did the procedures that were used. Before we share the optimism of both authors it seems that controlled replication of the entire investigation is called for.

Nevertheless, these procedures expand the compass of significant conditions, which we believe can be important for the outcome of therapy. We shall discuss several of these supplementary measures in the next chapter.

SUMMARY

A critical review of the first chapter on therapy warrants the following statements:

(1) *Short-term effects of treatment*: Up to this time no method of treating speech has proved to be unequivocally superior. There are hardly any long-term studies that currently support such a claim. For the most part, however, various procedures result in rapid immediate symptom reduction when first introduced, in many cases even to complete failure-free speech. It appears further that nearly all of the methods mentioned, at least according to reported long-term experience, remain effective only for a short period of time. In most clients for whom management has been confined only to speech, renewed short- or long-term deterioration sets in and results in far-reaching cancellation of the results of the procedures that have been introduced. When time and again great results are claimed for *new* procedures, we should view them with skepticism, at least until long-term studies are carried out (note especially comments on results of therapy and prognosis in Chapter 11).

(2) *Distinctiveness of treatment methods*: Many possibilities exist for influencing stuttering immediately and effectively. They offer the therapist broad opportunities to decide suitable procedures in each case based on their clients' individual characteristics and capabilities. However, in every case the stated goal is to lead the stutterer progressively back to a normal and fluent manner of speaking. If auditory self-control of speech and disturbances of central integration and coordination due to feedback interferences are the causal factors underlying the stuttering (as we assume in Chapter 4), then the therapeutic goal of most possible failure-free speech to be gained by use of aids to speech constitutes a hazard standing in the way of a successful outcome.

The immediate effectiveness of most methods is explained by a shifting of attention from the self-control of speech to other stimulus conditions (for example, pacing of speech by the beat of a metronome) or to other behaviors (for example, sign language). In the past such distracting mechanisms were employed in many therapies. In the eighteenth century itinerant physicians offered a magic remedy wherein the stutterer had to carry under his or her tongue a moistened wad of cotton rolled into a ball. That stuttering immediately disappears can easily be demonstrated with a lemon-flavored wad. However, as soon as the effect of the wad of cotton wears off the stuttering reappears. Another distracting mechanism, also used by therapists to this day, is the insertion of rhythmic movements of hands and arms, for example, using the right arm to describe the figure "eight" in the air. These two examples illustrate the possible short-term effectiveness of the methodology in treating speech.

The outcome is conceivably open to question since the stutterer (stimulated by the therapist) once having listened carefully to his or her "failure-free" speech, engages in an "evaluation" of the result. If the methodology does not also serve as a diversion, in part at least, then he or she quickly reverts to self-control of speech by feedback and, regrettably, to renewed failures. Furthermore, gradual habituation to the speech aid (that is, when it is no longer necessary to concentrate on this feature of the treatment method) also constitutes a predisposition to relapse. The client has in the meantime (and simultaneously) forgotten (or does not consider it necessary) to attend to it while talking. We shall return to this critical point when we consider the question of self-control (in Chapter 8).

(3) *The isolated use of a speech aid*: To understand what amounts to only short-term effects of speech aids we need to take into account, among other things, that in most of the studies the aids were used solely in isolation. Stuttering is, indeed, more than "only a disturbance of the speech mechanism" (Westrich, 1978, p. 2373). Stuttering manifests itself in the life experiences and behavior of the individual comprehensively and drastically. Therefore, in every case stutterers require correspondingly comprehensive and complex measures to alter their learning and living circumstances to accomplish their rehabilitation and not, or not only, treatment of symptoms (Westrich, 1978). The observation that the results of the procedures mentioned above hold only over the short term is basically due to the focusing of treatment exclusively on the speech of the stutterer and to indifference to other behaviors and experiences as well as to social determinants. We shall discuss this further in succeeding chapters.

We shall next present and discuss various measures that are recommended to support and supplement the treatment of speech.

Chapter 7

Measures Preceding and Accompanying Treatment of the Speech Disorder

INTRODUCTION

In previous chapters we presented various approaches to the modification of the speech disorder. It was made clear that these approaches were only relatively effective if they were not integrated into a comprehensive program that addressed the complexity of stuttering and took into account not only speech but its concomitant symptoms and the constraints on social interaction of the stutterer. An example just discussed is the "rapid therapy program" of Azrin and Nunn (1974).

However, before we go into detail concerning the practicability of an integrated complex therapeutic program (in Chapter 10) it is well to present and to evaluate separate aspects of other comprehensive approaches to treatment. These include approaches that have been proposed by several authors as supplements and extensions of exclusive speech training, such as improvement in the perception of one's own symptoms, the use of tape and video playback, attention to breathing, techniques of tension relaxation, as well as supportive medication for speech.

TRAINING FOR SYMPTOM AWARENESS (SELF-OBSERVATION)

Various authors view the improvement in competence to observe symptomatic behavior and to be discriminatively aware of its complexity as an important prerequisite to management of speech. This is done in diverse ways. Some have observed that stutterers are hardly able to report the moment of their stuttering accurately (for example, by pressing a signal button). However, they are quite able to *predict* the extent and locus of stuttering if the circumstances (locality, persons who are present, time of the day, especially "difficult" words, etc.) are known to them (Chapter 1). The aim of several authors in improving self-perception of stuttering immediately is to build up a realistic attitude toward it to counteract the "mystification" grounded in fearful and understandable expectations (Williams, 1957; Rieber, 1965; Van Riper, 1973). Clients actively need to adopt an attitude toward and come to terms with their symptoms so that they may come to know they are not exactly powerless in the face of their disturbance.

Other authors describe stuttering as a disturbance of perception (Cherry & Sayers, 1956; Yates, 1963a; Adams & Moore, 1972). The problem, as they see it, is that the disorder is indeed maintained when the stutterer devotes an excess of anxious self-control to his or her speech (related to its quality), which inevitably results in disturbance of coordination of speech due to possible interferences by auditory feedback. Therefore, as accompanying measures for speech therapy they recommend procedures for diverting the stutterer from his or her own speech difficulties, especially from differentiation between stuttering and not stuttering. These include shadow speech, insertion of white noise, and also paced speech and sign language. These are the prominent methods related to self-control of speech aimed at a kind of passive conquest of symptoms.

However, as has been shown by studies of negative practice (Widlak, 1977), controlled drilling and improvement in self-perception lead, though not inevitably, to reduction of symptoms. In many cases this can presumably be explained by a shift in the orientation of attentiveness brought on by the self-perception. The focus is no longer on the effort to achieve as symptom-free speech as is possible. Becoming acquainted with the symptomatology in all of its complexity is now the focal point. Mimicking and gesture are included here as well as attention to the effect of stuttering on interlocutors and their reactions to the experience and awareness of the client (see especially Van Riper, 1973, pp. 245–265). When such focus on symptom complexity has been assured, instruction in self-observation is introduced based on the proposition that stuttering is a consequence of interferences by auditory feedback growing out of perceptual defect. Our model is also based on this assumption. Active attention to complex conditions related to symptoms lessens the danger that attentiveness will be concentrated on the quality of speech. Here is where sign language methods particularly can be turned to good account.

Furthermore, the aim of enabling stutterers to achieve long-lasting self-control of their speech and to no longer have a need for therapeutic care requires them to know their complex symptom pictures as definitely as possible. This is an essential prerequisite for every kind of self-control, let alone for the quest for modification of self (see especially Chapter 8).

Children frequently associate questionable reactions to their stuttering on the part of parents with "illness" and "naughtiness." Along with training for self-observation, Schulze (1973) undertook cognitive reconstructions during therapy. Child and therapist listened together to a tape recording of the child's stuttering. They both shook a matchbox playfully whenever stuttering occurred in the child's utterances. After a short time the therapist dropped out and the child carried on alone. The author reported a case of a child in which this exercise led to marked "relief" due obviously to the changed attitude toward the disorder.

Perception of symptoms by self-observation can generally be achieved by voluntary stuttering or also with the aid of mirrors and tape or video recordings. In our own studies of treatment similar training using a recording was included. This involved reading, picture description, and free speech of varying degrees of difficulty in that order (Schmidt & Standop, 1974). Clients were told to indicate onset of a symptom by signaling with a flashlight. The aim of this exercise was to identify all symptoms as soon as possible. Then, only conspicuous behaviors closely associated with stutterings were similarly addressed. Later the exercises were further accommodated to awareness of internal as well as external conditions.

From the point of view of therapy it is wise to carry out this exercise as an independent entity *before* the introduction of speech techniques (Wendlandt, 1972), especially if the possibility of change in the client's attitude toward his or her symptomatology is assumed. We have also looked into this. In the next step identification of symptoms and then timely identification of occurrence of particular symptoms were recorded. The therapist then entered these directly onto a graph so that in the end the client saw displayed feedback of the results of the exercise. The exercise was terminated when more than 90% of all symptoms including difficult units were recorded.

A good point of reference in all of this was that the client found the training to be irksome. Because we were convinced that symptom reduction in our clients was due to this training we decided it would definitely be included in subsequent treatment. Interestingly, clients characterized awareness training as a "meaningful experience" through which they learned to view their symptoms differently from the way in which they had thought about them up to that time (Schmidt & Standop, 1974).

SOUND AND VIDEO RECORDINGS IN SPEECH THERAPY

The comments that follow are concerned with the feasibility of the use of video and sound recordings in developing new speech habits. Sound and video recordings are important, over and above this purpose, in social training, which will be discussed in Chapter 9. The use in therapy of visual and acoustic feedback of complex patterns of behavior has been extraordinarily effective in the past, especially in behavior therapy (Berger, 1970; Griffiths, 1974). Sound and video recordings have been mainly used to communicate objective information to clients (for example, only the verbal feedback of the therapist) concerning behavior problems and behavior changes in order to improve their discriminating skill and their potential for self-regulation and evaluation. It is rather surprising, indeed, that studies of the effectiveness of the use in stuttering therapy of video and sound feedback are virtually lacking.

Gregory (1968) indicated briefly that in his experience sound and video documentation of stuttering behavior was not entirely without its problems. Many clients expressed intense anxiety when the therapist sought permission for tape recording just for diagnostic purposes. Berger (1970) reported that this occurred in about 80% of other kinds of clients. The obvious problem for stutterers is that to have their difficulties, their helplessness and, in any case, their self-conscious gestural tensions fed back to them visually constitutes an especially tough and overpowering hurdle. Various studies suggest that self-confrontation and self-observation by video may impede therapy in the case of clients who suffer from a self-devaluing attitude (Zimmer, 1976). As we have seen, such an attitude fundamentally characterizes most stutterers. Is this basically enough to contraindicate the procedure?

In individual case studies we have sought to find conditions favorable for the use of magnetic tape recordings in treatment (Schmidt & Standop, 1974; Hofmann, Oertle, & Reincke, 1975). The comments that follow have grown out of those experiences.

The most important prerequisites to gain the participation of clients in the use of sound and video recordings appear to be choice of the right point in time and appropriate rationale for the introduction of the procedure in order to preclude negative effects right from the start. It is beneficial for clients to have acquired familiarity with the therapeutic task and with the procedures of the therapist beforehand—the overall "work atmosphere"—and for client and therapist to cooperate willingly. The technical apparatus should be familiar to them. We did not keep from our clients the information that video recordings would be made at the beginning of therapy under supervision of the therapist. From the beginning of treatment all clients learned to know recording techniques, transmission, and reproduction in a control room. One client expressed his desire to work with the video playback immediately after we explained at the first session that it was necessary and pertinent to his therapy. However, recordings for therapeutic purposes should first be made only if clients have made initial progress in other treatment modes.

Finally, before the first taping (recording of symptoms or in the context of therapy) is done it is a good idea to discuss the contemplated recording as it bears on the client's expectations and apprehensions. The aim should be to clear up potential verbalized client "resistance." Fundamentally, the therapist should make every effort to consider the arguments and the reservations of the client. The time course and the degree of difficulty of the planned training should be in accord with the client's willingness and capability.

To begin with, single recordings should not exceed a playing time of two or three minutes. Careful analysis of this time segment of tape can stretch out to as much as 30 minutes.

Once the recordings have been prepared the following procedures have been found to be practicable in discussing the video tapes (also correspondingly suitable for sound tapes) and how they can counter anticipated self-devaluation:

1. To begin with, the whole recording (two to three minutes) is viewed by client and therapist together. The two-to-three-minute time course should be strictly adhered to so that the client is not left "alone" for too long with potential thoughts of unpleasant life experiences. If for some reason the tape lasts longer, the discussion can be broken down into two or more segments.

2. After the first reproduction, reactions, reflections, feelings, etc., of the client engendered by the display of his or her behavior are ascertained. Here sufficient time and opportunity are also made available to allow the client to express unpleasant life experiences frankly, especially when he or she sees himself or herself on the screen for the first time. The therapist should express an interest in these statements. If problems and difficulties (later also progress) are perceived and verbalized by the client, the therapist should note as an aid to recall the point at which the client expressed the problem with a comment such as "We need to look more carefully at this once again." On the occasion of this first sketchy commentary the therapist should comment only if the client requests him or her to do so directly and if the client has reacted to the tape.

3. Detailed analysis of the comments about the tape follows. Here the entire tape is played back and gradually discussed in brief segments (15 to 30 seconds or even shorter). This is the sequence unconditionally adhered to: Viewing the tape together—description by client of what is seen and heard as well as his or her reactions—recording of

problems by therapist. Now, however, with every statement of a problem by the client a question is put by the therapist as to whether the described problem behavior is alterable (such as "Do you already have any idea how to get hold of this problem?" or "Can you envisage how you would change it next time?"). At this point the therapist can offer his or her suggestion. If it is at all possible the acquired changes in behavior are practiced immediately.

4. After this, several brief scenes are similarly discussed and if recommendations for changing problem behavior are being considered, the tape is repeated. In so doing the therapist not only takes care that the client does not undertake too much but also tries intensely to achieve vital behavioral changes. In this situation the therapist must carefully judge whether the repetition will result in recordable progress. This is necessary to motivate the client to continue cooperation.

5. Discussion of the tape follows the first repetition in a sequence exactly like the one following the initial presentation. Additional repetitions are recommended if time permits and if the client is not fatigued.

Such a procedure is useful if planning includes the use of video recordings to change mimicking, gesture, or sign language. Whether and to what extent viewing their symptoms should be demanded of clients varies from case to case. In making the decision, thought should be given to how much immediate progress is expected in treatment. Confronting video or sound tapes in therapy makes sense only if there is likelihood of improvement in symptomatic behavior.

The advantage of concentration on feedback from sound tapes is that they can be introduced sooner than video tapes. Moreover, discussion can be confined to an audible referent exclusively. Attention can be directed to speech variables such as loudness, intonation, pitch, and rate. Nevertheless, thought should be given to the possibility that these exercises may in the end cause clients to again orient themselves to intensified auditory self-control of their own speech. This could lead to questionable outcomes. It is important to use sound tape in speech training very carefully (Schmidt & Standop, 1974). Attention should not be focused on the symptoms but should concentrate on a definite training aim (for example, to read 100 bisyllables paced by a metronome). In practice, after final listening to the tapes the extent to which such requirements were met and the consequences for speech outside of therapy were reviewed. Schwartz (1977) found that there was evidence, for example, of a carryover to "normal" metronome-controlled speech. Schwartz also used sound recordings to verify the effectiveness of his "blowing" method for speech therapy (Chapter 6).

CONTROL OF BREATHING

In Chapter 1 we mentioned the observation that stutterers frequently breathe abnormally while talking. Downton (1956) compared the breathing of stutterers under four different conditions. One of his noteworthy single findings was that those stutterers who in the experimental situation were instructed to try to prevent their stuttering showed conspicuous irregularities in breathing. It may be that the genesis of stuttering and the development of abnormal breathing are related. Just as is the case with concomitant gestural and mimicking movements, altered breathing of stutterers may also be due to their attempts to overcome their speech difficulty. Moreover, abnormal inhaling or exhaling while talking may also develop. Long years of fruitless attempts to suppress symptoms can also lead to irregularities of breathing. At any rate, as Heese (1967) has found, this applies only to breathing while talking; breathing at rest generally is normal in stutterers. Arnold (1970b) reported additional observations. Schilling (1965) warned against mistakingly regarding abnormal respiratory function as a cause of stuttering.

The view that a fundamental modification of breathing can also achieve a reduction of stuttering has been variously advanced. However, the results thus far of including breathing therapy in the management of stuttering have been rather modest. Important in this connection are the observations that breathing gets to be normally regulated in the course of successful treatment of speech without any obvious direct assistance. Based on similar experience with children, Vlassova (1958) agreed with this.

Many authors have suggested that aberrant breathing may render speech training more difficult (Fernau-Horn, 1969; Azrin & Nunn, 1974; Schwartz, 1977). They therefore recommend purposeful drilling in new breathing habits as preparatory and supportive measures in speech therapy. This would foster, if not even accelerate, a manner of speaking incompatible with stuttering (Perkins, 1973a, b).

One of the most important requisites for regularity of breathing is considered to be sufficient intake of air prior to speaking (see the procedure of Azrin and Nunn, 1974, described in the preceding chapter). This applies especially to those who tend to talk with residual air and who speak many words as hastily as possible without a breath stop. Inspired speech is completely cut off. In considering "paradoxical breathing," drawing in the abdominal wall when breathing in and lifting and arching it forward when breathing out (Schilling, 1965), sequenced breathing exercises for proper speech training are advisable. Tunner (1973) looked into the feasibility of biofeedback to attain improved breathing. Clients saw their own breathing action through visual feedback by monitor. Their task was to try to achieve a regular continuous breathing curve (aided by this feedback) in paced speaking (speaking in synchrony with a metronome). However, to counter the loss of the control function of the visual feedback this had to be coupled with social and finally generalized reinforcers.

It is a good idea, especially in therapy with children, to introduce breath control measures in play form (see also Chapter 10). A disc recording by Berendes and Schilling (1962) offers an example of incorporating breath control measures inconspicuously.

The child plays a magician: "I am a great magician—shshsh—and I have two coins in my hand—shshsh—etc." The child associates each insertion of the "shshsh" sounds between each speech segment directly with the magic and does not interpret them as breathing exercises.

RELAXATION TECHNIQUES

It is easy to observe considerable diminution of agitation and tension in the general behavior of the stutterer during breathing exercises. In autogenic training (Schulz, 1969) as well as in progressive muscle relaxation (Jacobson, 1938) calm and deep inspiration and expiration are used to facilitate physiological relaxation. In speech therapy, too, calm, deep inspiration and slow expiration are used to reduce tension especially of the motor variety. In the therapy program of Azrin and Nunn (1974) inspiration and slow production of words were coupled with the self-instruction "I am completely calm and relaxed" to enhance the relaxing effect of breathing.

Controlled breathing and general motor relaxation can be combined with one another effectively. It is a good idea to do this preparatory to speech training if stutterers manifest extreme tension and parakinesis. Böhme (1966) makes several suggestions concerning this. In training sessions the stutterer should assume as "loose" a body posture as possible in a seated position. The hands should be placed lightly on the inner surface of the thighs. Shoulder regions should be as relaxed as possible and should be loosely movable. The therapist can determine the relaxed state of the client by noting the flexibility of movement of the shoulders.

Seeman (1969) suggests taking advantage of speech itself as a supplementary calming influence during breathing and relaxation exercises. According to him this can be accomplished while speaking by forming softly voiced vowels after each inspiration and sustaining them as long as possible to prolong phonation (compare this with the "blowing technique" described in the preceding chapter). This mitigates aversion to talking.

Here, we are reminded once again of the "metronome-conditioned relaxation" of Brady (1973), who after instructing the client in progressive muscle relaxation then went ahead with exercises in paced speech with the client relaxed (see Chapter 6).

Practical relaxation methods are usually recommended along with other measures for reduction of the motor stiffness that we see in almost all stutterers. This can be done by progressive muscle relaxation or by autogenic training. However, the latter method has several contraindications (for example, detectable cerebral damage), so that prior medical consultation is positively indicated. Several familiar relaxation methods are directed to the reduction of tension especially of muscles of the face, maxilla, and neck that are involved in speech. Dostálová (1974) proposed a modification of autogenic training concentrated particularly on relaxation of the speech musculature. Krech (1963) likewise suggested a modification of autogenic training that was specially developed for adult stutterers. McIntire, Silverman, and Trotter (1974) reported on the use of transcendental meditation as a possibility for general easing of tension.

Since relaxation measures alone hardly bring about changes in speech behavior their use in treating stuttering is appropriate only in conjunction with other types of procedures. Thus, Schulze (1978) always supplemented relaxing measures in those clients (in cases of anxiety of somatic origin) whose psychogalvanic skin resistance was reduced before intending and/ or talking. Easing of tension (elevated galvanic skin resistance) as well as agitation (lowered galvanic skin resistance) was fed back to clients by a wearable biofeedback device that facilitated voluntary relaxation. The author reported sustained symptom reduction when this kind of continuing self-monitored attempt to ease tension was used along with speech. Our model (Chapter 4) explains this. The demanding efforts required of clients to concentrate continuously on relaxation limit the possibilities for simultaneous vigilant control of the quality of speech since the auditory channel is used for biofeedback.

In the systematic desensitization developed by Wolpe (1958) relaxation procedures play an important role within a framework of anxiety management. In this procedure the client is requested to think about anxiety-provoking situations (*in-sensu* desensitization). By simultaneous performance of behaviors incompatible with anxiety (for example, muscle relaxation) the association between the anxiety stimulus and the anxiety is extinguished (for theory and practice of systematic desensitization see also Florin and Tunner, 1975). *In-sensu* desensitization has been frequently recommended in managing speech fears of stutterers and has been used in rather controlled fashion (Rosenthal, 1968; Jones, 1969; Brutten, 1969). However, several authors have questioned the effectiveness of *in-sensu* desensitization for treatment of stuttering. Since anxiety of stutterers also derives from social sources and because it is a problem of considerable complexity, graduated social training has been recommended for *in-vivo* desensitization (Walton & Mather, 1963; Boudreau & Jeffrey, 1973; Ingham & Andrews, 1973a) or, at least, a combination of an *in-sensu* and an *in-vivo* approach (Marks, 1969; Wendlandt, 1972). These references should suffice until we return in Chapters 9 and 10 to therapy for social phobias.

DRUGS AND SPEECH THERAPY

Schilling (1965) sent 550 questionnaires to professionals of differing theoretical orientation in various countries asking them which treatment of stuttering had proved most effective. A question was asked, among others, about their experience with drugs in treatment. Of the 112 usable answers received, 62.5% of the respondents recommended aid to speech therapy by drugs more or less definitely; 37.5% objected to their use. However, even among the group of advocates there were reservations. Schilling himself spoke out against drug therapy as the *only* kind of therapy and affirmed the use of drugs (as did most of the respondents) as only "adjunctive" within a complex pattern of treatment.

We, too, have reservations about recommending drug support in speech therapy. Above all, we see the danger that taking drugs can create a false impression in the stutterer that he or she will be cured or improved just by swallowing a pill. The need for the stutterer to cooperate actively in the relief of his or her speech disorder can be greatly diminished. Likewise, the anticipated placebo effects lasting only for a short time can lead to false conclusions and possibly to continuing recourse to drugs when relapses occur.

Evidence from investigations of the use of psychopharmacological substances aimed at amelioration of speech disorders indicates that the results are negligible and argues against recommendation of drug therapy (Winkelmann, 1954; Holliday, 1959; Kent, 1963; Schilling, 1965). Thus far, results of investigations in which drugs were used along with other training procedures have led to varying conclusions (Seeman, 1934; Doubek & Pakesch, 1957; Schilling, 1965; Arnold, 1970b; Beech & Fransella, 1971). Well-controlled investigations, particularly double blind and longitudinal studies, are lacking. Currently, the use of drugs is indicated only if along with stuttering there are additional psychosomatic illnesses that appear to require drug treatment. Strong indication is absolutely essential in every case. In such a case the therapist who is treating the stuttering should have a precise record of any possible side effects of drug treatment that can possibly negate his or her therapeutic efforts. This certainly can happen with psychopharmacological treatment (Linden & Manns, 1977).

SUMMARY

In this chapter we presented therapeutic measures that have been variously used preceding or accompanying speech therapy. Training for perception of symptoms as well as the use of video and sound recordings were noted. Specific indications for these measures were discussed and the problems and hazards associated with their use were delineated. The influence of breathing and relaxing techniques was generally considered to be beneficial. Drug support for speech therapy should be considered with great caution.

Chapter 8

Self-Control and
Self-Modification of
Stuttering

INTRODUCTION

In the preceding chapters the prerequisites and the possibilities for therapy with regard to speech disorders were presented and discussed. In the following sections we shall turn more directly to the question of how improvement in the speech of stuttering clients can be so maintained that lasting results can be anticipated. In recent years a great number of isolated investigations of the application of behavior therapy to a wide variety of behavior disorders have sought to demonstrate (and also have extensively documented) that the successful control of symptomatic patterns of behavior by the client himself or herself (so-called *self-control*) is the best precondition for long-term results (see especially Hartig, 1974; Mahoney & Thoresen, 1974; Thoresen & Mahoney, 1974; Kanfer, 1977; Meichenbaum, 1977). We shall try to determine the extent to which the potential of self-control carries over to the treatment of stuttering, particularly from the point of view of generalization of improvement in speech achieved in therapeutic sessions to situations outside of therapy.

Furthermore, if procedures in self-control learned in therapy are generally appropriate for facilitating transfer to the natural life circumstances of the client then the question now is how can the stutterer be guided to incorporate procedures to control and subsequently to change undesirable behaviors voluntarily. It is useful to look for an individually instituted form of self-management that enables the stutterer to activate behaviors that reduce and subsequently eliminate stuttering even in circumstances that are particularly difficult (so-called *self-modification*).

The case for self-control and self-modification presents a paradox if therapy is based on our previously stated assumptions about the origin and maintenance of stuttering (see Chapter 4). There we claimed that self-control of the quality of speech was responsible for the maintenance of the speech disorder.

If the client controls the quality of his or her speech auditorily then interferences over different feedback pathways (between kinesthetic and acoustic bone and air conduction channels) result in failures of integration that disturb speech coordination substantially and thus foster stuttering.

Here formidable problems arise not only for the use of technical forms of speech treatment, as we have seen, but also for attempts to achieve self-control of stuttering. The paradoxical situation that stuttering is occasioned by continuing attempts to avoid stuttering by self-control complicates therapy to an exceptional degree because all of the efforts of the stutterer, his or her caretakers, and possibly even former therapists are more or less open to question.

We believe that the following approach would be effective in dealing with this problem in therapy: It requires complete explanation to the client about the conditions for the origin and changing of the stuttering. The therapist pursues this course of action if the client is reasonably able to follow theoretical arguments. We shall propose a comprehensive model on this point and suggest arguments for discussion. An explanation of this kind facilitates winning the client over to the use of self-control procedures that make more difficult and even eventually prevent auditory monitoring. In our opinion, success in explanation is the route to self-modification of the speech disorder.

Generally, a plan involving the following sequence of steps is useful:

1. In therapy (specifically for youths and adults) explanation of the conditions of origin of and for changes in stuttering leads to a basis for therapeutic procedures.
2. Therapeutic intervention progressively expands the opportunities for self-control of stuttering.
3. Finally, the client is stimulated and guided to try out and to practice self-regulation in circumstances outside of therapy.

These steps will now be presented in detail.

THERAPIST AND CLIENT

Familiarizing average clients (youths and adults) with particular neuropsychological conditions that cause and maintain stuttering presents no problem. However, the explanation needs to be adapted to the language level and cognitive capabilities of clients to enable them to follow the arguments of the therapist.

A discussion such as this can determine whether the stuttering is possibly maintained by self-control of speech and whether this self-control is critically influenced by immediate demanding conditions. The interview data are helpful in making clear under what socially demanding circumstances the stutterer perceives himself or herself to have the severest difficulty in talking, when he or she is under greater strain in trying to talk fluently, and whether this strain is associated with improvement or, on the contrary, with more conspicuous stuttering. It is apparent that when the responsibility for communication is under slight or no pressure, speech comes easier and is more fluent if the client senses little or no fear of failure and perceives cognitively that self-control of speech appears to be less necessary.

The neuropsychological propositions are also demonstrated directly. We can have the client speak in the presence of white noise or paced by a metronome, for example, under conditions that make self-control difficult or under which external controls are superimposed on self-control. Additionally suitable for this are delayed auditory feedback (DAF), "shadow speech," and the introduction of various difficult circumstances such as speaking with the therapist while talking on the telephone. The therapist can refer to the difficulties associated with such conditions: after temporary success any therapeutic measure can lead to relapse or it may not even be properly responded to in the first place if the effort of the client is stubbornly fixed on the desire for success and on the notion that he or she will verify the results in speech behavior himself or herself. This dilemma brings up an extremely critical point, which demands great deftness and special sympathetic understanding on the part of the therapist. For it is essential that clients not concentrate their efforts on speech improvement even though in speech therapy this is their main concern and frequently that of their caretakers.

Therefore, it is crucial to introduce new goals for therapy, insofar as the therapist is able, in order to attain the objective "improvement of speech behavior and amelioration of stuttering." The client should be made to recognize that assigning primary importance to them makes good sense. Such "new" goals can be specified.

The client should be guided to more fluent speech employing procedures that make auditory self-control of speech more difficult or that replace it, more or less, with external stimuli.

The client learns to divert attention from the quality of his or her speech and direct it to various social situations requiring speech, as, for example, associating motor activity with speech (imitation and gesture); attending to the communicative signs of his or her interlocutor (imitation and gesture); concentrating on the subject matter of the conversation; focusing cognitively on the longer time course of a conversation, etc.

The client should learn to bring his or her influence to bear in social contexts actively (taking into account interlocutors, place, time, and organization of discourse).

Every one of these goals demands urgent attention of the client and they must be looked upon as contributing to an improvement in speech responsiveness. These goals guide the stutterer to voluntarily assign precedence to them over the need for auditory self-control of speech.

Since the client has presumably developed a reactive pattern (motor, affective, cognitive) to stuttering over a period of years this redirection of his or her attentiveness, activities, and behaviors cannot be expected to take place overnight. This should be obvious to the therapist right from the start; deep-seated patterns of reaction are not easily "erased." On the contrary, it is because of just such long-standing habits (with neurological correlates, called "Bahnungen" in German) that relapses can be expected. Therefore, planning for self-modification makes allowance for relapses since they are practically unavoidable. Here, too, the endeavors of the therapist to achieve cognitive restructuring are important. Relapses indicate to the client that the newly developed patterns of behavior are not sufficiently ingrained. Relapses urge caution. They should lead to a new phase of conscious self-control.

The recommendations and arguments that have been presented here can roughly demarcate the area in which the therapist can and should operate in his or her endeavor to accomplish the transition to self-regulation. They can motivate clients to shape their therapy actively. They differ from previous attempts at self-control in that the monitoring by clients of their own speech is less significant. In initiating attempts to achieve self-control in therapy it is essential to clarify the attitudes of stutterers toward their symptoms and, if need be, to change them by systematic explanation. The suggestions for implementing the proposals that have been made above can serve this purpose. That an objective and realistic adjustment to symptoms and to the difficulties of altering them can lead to better results and to more successful treatment has been variously reported (among others, Heese, 1967; Rieber, 1965; Sheehan, 1970d; Van Riper, 1973). Explanation concerned with causal factors and with substantiated evidence of conditions that foster change can also counter the "mystifying" of stuttering as an overpowering entity that keeps one helplessly in its clutches.

As a rule, stutterers have an extremely pessimistic view of the possibilities for altering their symptoms, especially following unsuccessful therapy. Many of their comments suggest that they see themselves as having succumbed to their symptoms (Frasier, 1956). For this reason, Schilling (1965) makes it emphatically clear to his clients that their speech organs are not damaged. He illustrates this during their intermittent fluent speech. He likens it to the case of the somewhat anxious driver of a car who steps on the brake in the face of oncoming traffic. The car stops. Yet he does not have an accident. This simple analogy also seems plausible to children. Hence Schilling works in the following key sentence at the beginning of therapy: "I do not have a speech disorder—no more than the car has engine trouble—I only step on the speech brake." Other illustrative descriptions and analogies are found in the work of Fernau-Horn (1969).

Just as Schilling, operating on the proposition that stuttering is a consequence of fear-generating circumstances, uses simple examples and illustrations to achieve cognitive restructuring, simple analogies certainly fit requirements of our model; for example, by retelling the familiar fable in which a cockroach asks a centipede how he is able to move his legs so elegantly and harmoniously. The centipede ponders the question and from that moment on can no longer walk. The development of problems for many stutterers is properly illustrated by this analogy. It is obvious that the all too cautious effort to avoid failure produces failure. It would indeed be difficult to avoid "compulsive self-control" in the future, not the least because increasing circumstances within social settings have taken on a powerful behavior-influencing function.

Conditions for Successful Self-Control

It is clear that the conditions for the introduction of measures to achieve self-control can be arranged within the basic framework of the ideas previously advanced. For some, aids to speech should be sought that (1) divert the attention of the stutterer from concentration on his or her speech activity to a stronger focus on other aspects of the communication situation and that (2) can be used and maintained by the client (also at the termination of therapy) without the therapist (self-control). For others, the possibilities that facilitate self-modification and provide long-term support should be explored. Here, care is taken to examine whether and how the measures that are used can be carried over to environmental situations and whether and how these have been applied by the client himself or herself. We shall next confine ourselves to addressing the first topics. A later section and a substantial portion of the following chapter will be devoted to the latter questions.

Aids to Speech

The claims for treatment procedures aimed at the relief of speech disorders that have been presented need to be scrutinized as to the extent to which they can be applied by clients themselves and can continue to be used independently.

To begin with there are the procedures that exploit the masking effect (white noise) and delayed auditory feedback (DAF). These have been shown to be anything but suitable for helping the client maintain the benefits over the long term. Yet, they are very appropriate now and then as a step in speech therapy. Sooner or later, however, supplementary procedures are required that enable the transfer of new modes of speaking learned under masking or DAF conditions. Likewise, the method of negative practice cannot be carried out by clients themselves. These methods are only starting points for more broadly designed therapy.

In the same way stimulus sources such as metronomes, haptometronomes, and micronomes serve only as preparatory means for establishing a new mode of speaking and are gradually faded out. Continued use through acquisition or construction of these devices by the client himself or herself is advisable only in exceptional cases; for example, in cases of extremely severe disorders when the device appears to be significantly helpful to the client and he or she does not want to dispense with it. Shadow speech and simultaneous speech, of course, are dependent on help and monitoring by another person. Also, even if training is possible without a partner (for example, by talking along with a radio or tape recorder), it can hardly be considered a significant method outside of therapy. What remains is the introduction of recommended speech training procedures (sign language, possibly blowing techniques, as well as additional breathing exercises) that require self-responsibility as early as possible for their continuance outside of therapy. We shall go into these latter possibilities again in greater detail.

Self-Control Through Speech Training

Gesture language as a medium in therapy is particularly suitable as a possible first step in training for self-control because it can be combined with other speech training procedures (for example, the blowing technique) as well as with speech aids (especially with shadow and simultaneous speaking and paced speech), or it can be a useful adjunct to them. This permits progressive advances and systematic controllable practice in new speech habits. Also, consistent with the propositions of our model, it is possible by means of gesture language to attain beneficial diversion of attention from self-monitoring of the quality of speech to other more important aspects of the speech act and of communication circumstances.

How then can the client be guided to cognitively controlled (i.e., voluntarily self-directed) monitoring of his or her gesture language?

To begin with, features of gestures can be emphasized. The attention of the client should be drawn to the movements of arms and hands as nonverbal support of the spoken word. Then, body postures (upper body, movements of the trunk, positions of the head and legs, manner of sitting and standing, self-initiated movements) can be associated with speaking. Other exercises are soon feasible that should encourage the stutterer to make the effort to redirect his or her concentration on speech output to focus on other thoughts. Attention should be directed more and more to the content and less to the quality of what is said. Free expression (as, for example, in describing objects in the therapy room or telling of pleasant experiences) and narration of fairy tales can serve as beginning exercises, just as carefree games and creative activities can draw greater attention to themselves during speech than can simple description. We ask questions that stimulate free association (such as, "What are all the things that can be made of cardboard?"). In going through these procedures we must constantly observe whether the client searches for appropriate gesture language that functions as help and nonverbal illustration for the spoken word and then uses it even though it does not ideally fit the spoken word in every case.

We have observed that intentional concentration on the content of spoken language in order to make the self-monitoring of speech output more difficult is not sufficient in every case to result in fluent speech. This may be due, among other reasons, to the notion that the train of thought giving rise to speech can be interrupted when the stutterer talks. Attention can easily be directed to speech production (as an expression of habit). More fluent speech is attainable only by making habitual self-monitoring of speech more and more difficult, as is done with continuing and conscious use of speech gestures.

Further along in training, systematic focusing of attention on other aspects of communication can be achieved. The stutterer can learn to ask himself or herself questions similar to the following (and answer them):

How well have my interlocutors taken in what I have said? What can I read in their faces? What does their nonverbal behavior, their gestures tell me? Where do they direct their gaze when I speak? Do they look at me? Are they pleased with what I say? Does it make them thoughtful? Or sad? Do I sit and stand properly? Or should I change my posture? etc.

During therapy sessions the client asks similar questions in a loud voice over and over again. Answers to such questions are spoken loudly. Such "loud" practice of new "trains of thought" is worthwhile not only because the learning effects and practice in new ways of thinking become known to the therapist but also because the client, compelled to speak slowly, cannot easily or quickly "think away" this new way of reflecting.

In the exercises that have been described, blowing techniques, additional breathing drills, as well as relaxation procedures can be included beneficially (see Chapters 6 and 7). Recall the "fundamental alteration in speech habits" referred to by Azrin and Nunn (1974), the effects of which are traceable, certainly in large part, to redirection of attentional habits. There is a relation between their procedures and training in using gestures associated with speech.

The need to divert clients from monitoring of the quality of their own speech was recognized as early as the first half of this century in many concepts of therapy based on diverse theoretical points of view. Interestingly enough, this is evident in the work of authors who are themselves stutterers or who were stutterers in their youth. For example, Hoepfner (and Meyer, 1926), who until late adolescence was himself a stutterer and had spent a long time in residence in a speech clinic, gave such pointers as these to teachers and caretakers of stuttering children: Be consistent in disregarding the stuttering and do not persist in "drills" because the child can be made thereby to concentrate on his or her speech failures; the word "stuttering" should never be used; the stutterer must let his or her speech flow automatically and not let it be governed by conscious regulation; a changed manner of talking can provide for more fluent speech. As early as the middle of the last century, C. Wyneken (1868), also a stutterer, held a similar point of view. Explanation to the stutterer concerning the possibilities for changing symptoms constituted one of the fundamental bases of his therapy: "We must remove doubt from the stutterer and do all we can to replace it with confidence, i.e., belief in his own ability" (p. 21). Wyneken had already recommended procedures that today still number among our important helpful interventions, namely, aid in breathing and paced speech.

IMPLEMENTATION AND TESTING OF SELF-MODIFICATION

For appropriate trials of techniques developed for self-control we suggest the following procedures which can mediate long-term competency in self-modification:

(1) *Probing the usefulness of self-control techniques*: Concrete situations are sought in which timely practice of self-control learned in therapy is feasible. These are delineated as specifically as possible (time, place,

interlocutor, and other social circumstances). The question here is what circumstances can occur that may aggravate probing of the natural environment or may even prevent it? In using his or her newly learned strategies for surmounting difficulties, it may be necessary, perhaps, for the client to deal with failures actively as well as cognitively.

(2) *Availability*: In an actual training situation we make certain that the client is really prepared to carry out his or her newly developed behaviors. At the end of a therapy session a careful summary of intended purposes (for example, available protocols) is often sufficient. It is a good idea now and then to put into writing carefully thought out sequences of actions, details of situations agreed upon in training sessions, expected successes and incidental failures and counterstrategies to prevent failure. This is usually done in that part of the therapy session when various topics are being discussed and toward the end of the session when the client may show signs of training fatigue. The client takes such a written piece home (for overlearning, so to speak), reads it through several times a day, and carefully and repeatedly prepares himself or herself. Contracts between client and therapist are suggested to strengthen the obligation of agreements. Entering into these kinds of "sociable" agreements frequently presents the client a better opportunity once more to finally overcome his or her existing fears and to dare to "leap into the cold water." (For structured use of therapeutic contracts, see Kanfer, 1977.)

(3) *No fear of failure!* It is helpful for the client to develop a cognitive readiness to tolerate social failure. Such readiness can be motivated by the possibility that discussion of the circumstances of failure can undoubtedly contribute to more precise steps in planning and training. Constant avoidance of situations in which failure may be anticipated only makes it very difficult to include specific activities since no concrete experiences are available. Improvement of social and communicative competence through training is only provisionally possible and does not guarantee that success will follow later (also Chapter 9). Avoidance of difficult situations also precludes the potential unexpected experience that can be handled relatively well or is even completely satisfying.

Fundamentally, self-monitoring is due, in large part, to the fear of stuttering. Out of fear of exposing themselves stutterers constantly seek to conceal their stuttering and this fear alone perpetuates self-monitoring and with it, stuttering. Perhaps the stutterer can break this vicious circle by immediately making known publicly that he or she is a stutterer instead of revealing it by stuttering: "It is somewhat difficult for me to talk; despite this, I shall speak because what I have to say is important!" If the interlocutor knows that the client is a stutterer then the ill-fated efforts to avoid exposing himself or herself as a stutterer will be subverted. If this is a decisive variable, and there is much to be said for it, then such a forward step greatly reduces intensified subjectively experienced communication responsibility (and with it a diminution of the stuttering follows). A step toward "open revelation of stuttering" such as this is a central element in Sheehan's Role Therapy (1970d). Schwartz (1977) offers his clients wearable buttons that say "I stutter occasionally, therefore I talk slowly."

(4) *Motivation for self-modification*: Various authors have referred to the difficulty of motivating clients to do "home" training exercises (Richter, 1972; Tunner, 1974). This is understandable. For almost all of their lives stutterers have constantly taken pains to discipline themselves. Caretakers have constantly demanded "correct" speech from them. Discernible results have for the most part failed to appear despite persistent effort. What is more, contrary and symptom-fixing effects may occur frequently. Nevertheless, the therapist should not avoid initiating attempts at self-management and should not forego efforts to continue extension of the self-therapeutic competence of clients if he or she wants to prepare them adequately for the risky posttherapeutic period. An important assist in motivating independent practice is to get the client to understand the quantitative difference between modest practice demands and self-induced fatigue. Furthermore, it should be made clear that therapeutic success cannot be expected if the newly learned patterns of behavior are manifested only during the therapeutic session. There is just no guarantee that some way or another everything on the outside will go smoothly. The therapist should express his or her judgment openly and candidly on the prognosis for treatment, not in any way that fosters resignation but in a manner that strengthens motivation by referring to conditions that contribute to a favorable prognosis (Chapter 11).

(5) *The necessity for control*: Attempts at self-modification utilizing the measures that have been described above assume a need for most careful supervision. However, it is difficult for the therapist to monitor a planned project outside of therapy. But in succeeding therapeutic sessions it is hoped that he or she will make concrete suggestions for change and improvement in explorations for self-modification. The hoped-for help from the therapist is facilitated by careful self-monitoring on the part of the client. This is more likely to occur if easily learned self-observation is practiced during therapy and meticulous protocols are kept. Both measures are also necessary for documentation of outcomes of therapy.

(6) *Self-observation*: The behaviors and the social conditions to be observed are determined precisely together with the client. In each case this depends, as a rule, on the self-control activities that have been practiced in therapy and on the goals of self-modification. Observation of the transfer effect can be accomplished to the extent that the client actively

and cognitively applies and voluntarily controls the various new features of his or her communication behavior. The client should ask these questions as soon after the try-outs of self-control as possible: (1) How successful have I been in using the behaviors that I have undertaken? (This question needs to be answered only if therapist and client have previously determined a criterion, lesser or greater maximum demand, for change in behavior.) (2) Why have I been successful with some and not with others? (Such an evaluation may be concerned with both voluntary active-cognitive issues and circumstances of the communication situation such as place, time, interlocutor, etc.) (3) Do immediate possibilities already occur to me for improving my conduct in the future under similar circumstances?

(7) *Protocols*: Immediate recording of protocols facilitates later evaluation of performance in self-control. Protocols should be in a form that is easily understood by the client. Prepared observation protocols can be recorded so that answers on the above questions can be incorporated in graphic or in some other simple form (for example, pinpoints). Keeping of protocols should be practiced together with the client so that difficulties in handling them can be cleared up beforehand. Furthermore, protocols should be continually subject to change with experience if, for example, simplification is indicated or a more complex form of presentation is useful.

(8) *Evaluation*: As long as therapeutic support continues the therapist should supervise and evaluate the steps taken by the client toward self-modification. This should take place at the beginning of every therapy session in order to try out purposeful necessary and feasible changes in the program of self-modification. Nevertheless, the objective of self-help measures is to make the therapist increasingly superfluous. This means that clients must master procedures for self-evaluation of self-modification and guided by these evaluations undertake changes independently and on their own responsibility. Here the therapist can give timely encouragement, for example, by asking the client during the therapy session to undertake changes in the program if these appear to be reasonable. Actual changes in behavior are planned and accomplished not only in the session but their concrete and flexible use is anticipated above all in the increasingly longer periods between sessions. Here, attention should be paid to adequate self-reinforcement. Kanfer (1977) suggests that individuals measure their performance based on norms that they themselves have established. The resulting rewards are thereby dependent on the "self-reinforcing pattern" of the involved person. Hence, therapy should endeavor to influence self-established norms and to encourage the kind of self-criticism by the client that leads to appropriate self-reinforcement.

SUMMARY

As the next chapter on management of social problems will show, programs directed to control of environment have their recognized limitations. For this reason it is important that ways be found along with the clients that enable them as soon as possible to feel comfortable in their relation with their therapist. In this chapter opportunities and problems of self-control and self-modification of stuttering were considered. It was generally recommended that

- the client be familiarized with the conditions that bring on stuttering in order to make clear the basic relations between them and the choice of treatment procedures
- treatment modes be sought for which the client is himself or herself responsible and which can also be used between therapy sessions
- these forms of self-management be practiced enough to ensure their generalization
- opportunities are introduced for self-monitoring during therapy so that they finally are carried on independently.

In this chapter we have only touched upon the therapeutic possibilities that effectively confront the more complex social determinants of stuttering with an attitude of self-responsibility. Therefore, we shall devote the next chapter to the treatment of social disorders.

Chapter 9

Treatment of Social Disorders

INTRODUCTION

If we glance back at the introductory chapter to this book we find continuing reference to the proposition that stuttering is not only a disturbance of speech but also always involves an array of impairments of the social competence of the stutterer. Before long the speech disorder causes stutterers to withdraw increasingly from social situations since they consider themselves "troublesome," as outsiders, and incompetent for many purposes. Later many avoid normal participation in social activities completely. In its wake the history of long-standing symptoms obviously brings on a condition in which adolescent and adult stutterers no longer share in normal social development. The stutterer learns social behavior under difficult conditions, much of it only by observation. He or she rarely has the opportunity to try out required social skills, to say nothing of using them. Gaps in knowledge appear. The result is a lack of appropriate social competence to deal with many communication situations and demanding circumstances. Disorders in social behavior are inevitably added to the speech disorder.

We would expect stutterers to endeavor to overcome the behavioral gaps and deficits that originate in the manner described above. But they just do not have the necessary competence to do so. Apparent allowances for their behavior made by caretakers make it impossible for stutterers to attempt the required adjustments in their behavior because constructive and essential social feedback is lacking. This leads ultimately to the development of inadequate modes and habits of behavior. It can therefore be confidently stated that the longer stuttering continues, indeed, the earlier it begins, the more likely are knowledge gaps, competency deficits, and the prevalence of anxiety and associated inadequate modes of behavior to persist. They then aggravate or prevent functioning in socially demanding situations.

Difficulties of this kind cannot be overcome if therapy is concentrated on treatment of the speech disorder only. We do not agree that during the course of treatment preparation for adequate social behaviors will "automatically" take place in most cases by chance or by the efforts of the stutterers themselves. The opposite happens more frequently. Although they may be talking fluently stutterers may turn away from social demands because they lack other appropriate behavioral competencies. It is certainly understandable that their social floundering will cause stutterers to withdraw and even to begin to stutter again in order, perhaps, to have socially acceptable grounds for failure. If, however, stuttering in this sense can be judged a social "illness," then modes of behavior of the individuals who comprise the contacts of the client need to be included in therapeutic thinking. Just as important are the consequences of symptom change for caretakers who may be responsible for the client in the future and for those individuals who are involved in interpersonal relations with him or her. There are many reasons for always including caretakers as much as possible in social therapy of stutterers.

Moreover, thought must be given to the likelihood that communicative and interactive practices developed in therapy may be established under relatively unrealistic conditions. The therapist may exhibit modes of behavior that are rarely ever encountered in real life (for example, indulgent listening, avoidance of cutting the stutterer short or completing a sentence for him or her, maintenance of eye contact and continuation of the conversation in the face of withdrawal tendencies on the part of the client). The therapist generally acts in a permissive, understanding, and patient manner, even when making demands, in order to give the client the opportunity for anxiety-free, conversational expression. However, despite the best intentions of the therapist, this prevents successful transfer. Thus, in the following sections we again raise the question as to how to arrange the therapeutic situation to facilitate the generalization of results achieved in therapy to everyday real-life conditions.

GENERAL REQUIREMENTS FOR POSITIVE TRANSFER

The success of therapeutic endeavors stands or falls on the transfer of training experiences to social conditions outside of therapy (Sieland & Schäuble, 1976). We have already devoted a good deal of attention to this fact in the preceding chapter on self-modification. Briefly, these are the preconditions for a successful outcome: (1) positive preparation of the client for new learning (enhancement of motivation), (2) making available necessary information (expansion of knowledge), as well as (3) developing command of required skills (expansion of social competence). Since access to realistic life situations may be difficult, the client is increasingly encouraged to accomplish transfer on his or her own.

In the following we shall present possibilities that facilitate generalization of therapeutic outcomes to natural situations and particularly to those that foster appropriate social behavior. They all aim to achieve lasting outcomes of therapy or, at least, to increase their probability.

CONSTRUCTING HIERARCHIES OF SITUATIONS MARKED BY ANXIETY

If it has not been done previously in the course of analysis of behavior (Chapter 5), it is necessary early in therapy to begin to organize social determinants of the stuttering in an orderly fashion to enable the proper choice and sequence of treatment steps in specified areas. To this end the client prepares a list of social conditions and rank orders them according to the degree of difficulty (for example, in talking) and, consequently, the anxieties that they generate. Situations that the stutterer handles rather well head the list, followed by those that present moderate difficulty. The inventory terminates with those situations that the stutterer no longer currently seeks out because the fears that he or she will not be able to endure them are most intense. Also several hierarchies can be simultaneously constructed concerned with various life and problem areas (for example, a hierarchy of situations in work places, communication·behavior in familiar and friendly circles, etc.).

The following plan for concrete measures in and outside of therapy refers to such hierarchies continuously. They allow for progressive steps forward and prevent steps that are too large. Specific aids to the construction and initiation of hierarchies are to be found, among others, in Morris (1977) and Florin (1975) and for particular use in stuttering therapy in Wendlandt (1972) and Van Riper (1973, pp. 270–273). Items of the hierarchy based on experience and the growth of competency of the client are rearranged continuously in the course of therapy. Regular review of the hierarchy is therefore necessary.

ROLE PLAYING

Role playing is a method especially familiar to behavior therapists. It affords a targeted systematic plan for modification of social anxieties and communication disorders. Everyday social conflicts of clients can be simulated in the therapy room in a practical way. These simulations aim to extend social deportment and competence. In the case of the stuttering client he or she learns to develop interests, wants, and desires, to reflect them to the interlocutor, and, if need be, to assert himself or herself against the therapist. Role playing has the potential for facilitating instruction in sensitivity to social relations as well as in realistic evaluation and proper use of one's own competencies. Role playing is suitable for preparation and try-out of self-modification.

Preparation and Implementation

As an example, training in social competence of stutterers can encompass the following steps (here we draw on experience in our own therapies; see also Chapter 10):

(1) *Delimiting the problem*: After construction of a hierarchy of difficult situations a decision about a problem area drawn from the hierarchy follows. The rank order of individual conditions therein listed roughly determines the procedures and the goals of the therapeutic activities. Then, the specific setting (time, place, potential interlocutor, other contexts) is determined for an item out of the chosen hierarchy (starting with an item that is associated with the least anxiety and gradually approaching the more stressful ones). Several contiguous items or items involving one another may be addressed together.

Illustration: It is evening, two brothers sit together at a table; both are drinking tea and nibbling cookies; radio music in the background; relaxed atmosphere. They engage in conversation typical for this situation, about current politics, family matters, work and profession, common familiar things, etc. This is an item out of the hierarchy that hardly gives rise to anxiety.

(2) *Concretization of the problem*: The problems encountered by the client under circumstances of the selected item are once again worked out and are specified at various behavioral levels (talking, experience, social communication, ability to interact, etc.).

Illustration: All of the above-mentioned conversational themes discussed in the presence of the brother were not deemed to be stressful. However, up to this point the client always expected his brother to initiate the conversation, although once it got under way the client talked rather effortlessly, somewhat like the way he talked to the therapist during therapy.

(3) *Concretization of solutions*: A decision then follows as to appropriateness of behavior or for a sequence of actions that lead to better coping

with the problem or to a reasonable solution to stated problems. In practicing interaction, sentences and sentence fragments that are likely to apply should be specified. These are spoken in accordance with the state of speech therapy at that time. Breathing behavior can be involved and gestures to accompany speech are determined beforehand. Gradually, many other aspects of treatment that make talking more difficult can be included.

Illustration: The client learns to initiate the conversation with his brother. For this he selects "current politics" as the practice theme; he can discuss an item with his brother that he has just read in the newspaper. An introductory sentence is formulated: "Fred, listen, I have just read ----." This sentence has been selected in order to obviate the use of a "starter" by client such as "I would like to say ----." Besides, the name of the brother (Fred) was placed at the start because during the discussion it was regularly stuttered (tonic at the beginning of words) by pressing the upper row of teeth against the lower lip. As he proceeds to initiate the conversation, the client puts the newspaper down and looks at his brother. Before speaking he once again takes a deep breath and begins to speak in a gentle voice ("blowing"). He points to the news item with the index finger of the right hand (avoiding finger snapping) and then moves his hands in concert with the speech (this has already been drilled on with him).

If the "difficult" words (i.e., those that are conspicuously stuttered) are ascertainable they are incorporated gradually in exercises (see also the reading exercises recommended by Brutten and Gray, 1961).

(4) *The arrangement of the room*: The therapy room should be arranged so that role playing (or other problem-solving activities) can be carried out undisturbed. Possible role-playing partners need to be chosen and included in the planning. It is a good idea to devote a session now and then exclusively to planning for those people involved in room arrangement or as participants in role playing who need basic preparation and to carry out the role playing in a subsequent session (after that, other participants will be found and they too can be similarly prepared in role-playing behavior).

For example, table and chairs can be so arranged that the therapy room is similar to a room at home. The therapist assumes the role of interlocutor (the brother). A daily newspaper is provided. Preparation is made for sound recording (microphone on the table).

(5) *Implementation of role playing*: Role playing is now ready to be carried out. It is important to emphasize to the client that this is a *training* situation and mistakes may be made. Repetitions and additional training are likely to be needed. As soon as the main factors in problem-solving behavior and the actions related to them have been successfully mastered in role playing, the exercise is terminated. Generally, duration of the

episode should not exceed five minutes, ensuring avoidance of fatigue and with it of experience of failure . Usually, rather short performances suffice for try-outs of new modes of behavior (one to two minutes). The shorter the performances the more likely are the repetitions. These broaden the opportunities for learning. If the therapist does not participate (as role-playing interlocutor), then he or she functions as a helpful stage director who is deliberately supportive from the sideline but is also demanding of the players throughout the performance.

We can expect, if the episode lasts two minutes, during which several phrases are exchanged between client and "brother" relating to a news-paper clipping spontaneously chosen by the client, that the client might stutter somewhat more conspicuously than during the planning phase of the performance.

(6) *Discussion of the performance*: Immediately after the conclusion of the episode the client should be given the opportunity to express freely what he felt and experienced during the performance. After this there is a general, and later a more detailed, analysis of the tape recording of the performance. The analysis essentially follows the steps recommended for discussion of sound and video recordings in Chapter 7. If no recordings are available the discussion must depend essentially on the recollections of the participants and any observer who may have been present. As a rule, this is far more difficult and less effective.

For example, the client indicates that the play was not as tough an experience as he had really anticipated; at the same time he also expresses misgivings about his ability to repeat the play in the same way at home. But in discussion of the sound tapes one gets the distinct impression that in several places the client spoke rather nervously and with residual air.

(7) *Repetition of the play*: One or more repetitions of the play follow. Formally, this should lead to planning for improvement in the problem-solving actions of the client (possibly of the interacting partner too) as described under points 3 and 4. Here, special emphasis is given to those aspects to which the client should pay attention during the repetition.

For example, should the client pay special attention to his breathing? Should he breathe in quietly before each sentence or long passage? After the intake of air should he make an effort to speak short sentences? Two more short repetitions follow.

It is essential to clarify the behavior of the "natural conversational partner" before the performance and subsequently to ascertain the extent to which the repeated play was "genuine."

(8) *Preparation for transfer*: Careful planning for transfer of skills learned in therapy concludes training in the selected item area. Place, time, and more detailed circumstances for a trial outside of therapy sessions are

determined precisely and the most important aspects of behavior are stressed once more.

Experience in role playing is also a beneficial prerequisite for testing practiced activities in critical circumstances. Careful planning of role playing is necessary to justify this claim. The therapist must judge beforehand whether the desired changes in behavior can really be achieved in the training session. Experience has shown that many performances of plays are frequently necessary before the client feels secure enough to really test out what has been learned. This needs to be taken into account in overall planning of the timing schedule of therapy. Hence, in the course of social training several sessions are scheduled to follow one another after short intervals (for example, daily sessions for a week).

Additional Comments

"Ascent" in the hierarchy to the next more difficult item area should take place only if the steps accomplished in therapy have been passed in crucial situations. Unfortunately, this is not always possible because problem situations do not conveniently appear "on call." If an immediate test of an "emergency" is not possible, careful planning of other procedures can compensate; for example, choosing an area for the next stage that ensures the testing of newly learned behavior in the context of everyday living.

After conjoint preparation for role playing by therapist and client many clients manifest modes of behavior soon after the first attempt that may have been inadequately specified. These behaviors indicate that the client still does not have command of appropriate ways of reacting to the selected problem situation. Stutterers may behave insecurely, hesitatingly, and even aggressively, feel rejected (in role playing too), react irritably, and be easily offended. These kinds of reactions usually slip into the behavior of stutterers and create additional difficulties for effective communication along with the speech problem. In many situations clients are often conscious of the inadequacy of their behavior. When discussing steps in social training the therapist along with the client should identify these disturbing behaviors carefully, should look for alternatives, and try them out in role playing and in everyday situations. Clients are not able on their own to execute particularly new and unfamiliar modes of behavior right off. Here a pretended appropriate behavior model can help significantly. Usually, the therapist functions as the model. In group therapy (see below) other clients demonstrate model behavior. It is remarkable how an appropriate model of complex behavior patterns of a client can be reproduced immediately. The potential for wide application of learning by model makes it especially effective as a strategy for change in all forms of role playing (Friedman, 1971; Eisler, Hersen, & Miller, 1973; Wendlandt, 1977).

In Chapter 7 we commented on the possibility of recording role playing performances on video tapes and using them as a basis for systematic discussion in training. The arrangement and the follow-up using video tapes of role playing in training is similar in principle to the procedures that have been described.

Training via role playing can help in carrying through one's own wishes, demands, and interests in varying social situations. Training in self-assertiveness can be used successfully to reduce the social fears of stutterers (Marks, 1969; Wendlandt, 1974). In between there is a whole array of activities for the initiation and implementation both in form and substance of self-training in assertiveness. We therefore limit ourselves to information on various activities involving the German language which the therapist can draw on as useful references in organizing therapy (Wendlandt & Hoefert, 1976; Flowers, 1977; Ullrich de Muynck & Ullrich, 1977; and Wendlandt, 1977).

Group Work with Stutterers

Role playing to advance social competence and self-training in assertiveness can also be carried out profitably in therapy groups. After progress in individual treatment has been made consideration needs to be given to whether and how group treatment should be offered. Continuation of therapy in a group allows for controlled use, under rather stressful conditions, of behavior competencies developed by the client in individual treatment. Several additional advantages are given by Wendlandt (1972).

The group situation enables clients to acquire the insight into their speech impediment that they are not alone in their difficulties and that others have likewise to make an effort to achieve changes in behavior. New modes of social behavior can be developed in the group without having to be simulated or introduced by the therapist. The group is an efficacious corrective of inadequate behavior since feedback concerning acquired modes of behavior by various individuals is provided repeatedly. It affords a variety of possibilities for learning by imitation and observation. This fosters the development of complex behavior patterns, especially if individual members of the group share their cognitive strategies (self-instruction, tactics, etc.) aimed at achieving designated objectives. The group provides a broader learning base since it functions as an important intermediate step to positive transfer. Social training situations should definitely not be contrived laboriously. The group itself is counted on continually as a training ground for social skills. Through conversation stutterers can be led to active (rational as well as emotional) analysis of their symptomatology, to attitudes about their problems, and to possibilities for self-identification and self-assertiveness. For general possibilities and problems involving systematic group management, see especially Lieberman (1977), Grawe (1978), and Fiedler (1978b).

TRANSFER OF TRAINING

The attainment of effective transfer definitely depends on the extent to which stutterers are enabled to transfer *gradually* to their own social milieu what they have learned in therapy. Steps that are too large and too demanding can result in failures and lead to relapses, possibly even to discontinuance of therapy. Fashioning demanding circumstances that approach reality as well as conjoint seeking out of everyday situations constitute a necessary condition for transfer of therapy. An essential first step is to arrange early and continuing participation in the therapy by strangers (for example, colleagues of the therapist, assistants, other co-workers, and also other stuttering clients). This takes place as early as during the first session of speech training. Modes of behavior and the number of participants are varied regularly and their manifold opportunities for practice are cleverly woven into speech therapy. Of course, it is important for the stutterer to declare that these measures are agreeable to him or her. We have already carried out several therapeutic training projects in the presence of twenty students and in so doing have correlated speech therapy with the hierarchy item of social therapy "speaking publicly before more than ten persons."

Soon after preliminary practice in therapy "therapeutic excursions" are undertaken. For example, we have often visited the market with clients and had them first engage in practiced shopping talk with clerks about the quality of their wares and then had them chat with housewives about the preparation of dishes. We also visited cafés and busy pubs in which conversation was engaged in with a waiter or persons who were seated at the same or a nearby table. All of this critical practice provides the therapist with an opportunity to witness speech and interpersonal habits that do not show up in therapy. Time and again, this has given us a chance to reconsider and simultaneously to correct transfer circumstances that we had arranged.

THE ROLE OF CARETAKERS IN THERAPY

The most beneficial prerequisite for successful transfer is to involve caretakers in therapy. This affords the possibility of gaining direct influence on those conditions that contribute considerably to the maintenance of stuttering and that stand in the way of effective therapeutic measures, especially when the stuttering clients themselves are not able to exercise much influence. Direct involvement of caretakers must be carefully thought out and planned. Agreement and understanding of the client and the involved persons are essential.

Participating caretakers are informed just as the stutterer himself or herself has been about the causes and the conditions required for change of the stuttering. This facilitates pertinent change in their adjustment to stuttering and to the client. In this "protected" therapeutic context stutterers can speak face to face more freely with their caretakers about their difficulties and problems just as the caretakers have the opportunity to describe their experiences as part of the environment of the stutterer. Relevant exchange of information as well as common exploration for possibilities for change constitute a cornerstone for profound alteration in the interpersonal relations between them.

In a restricted sense participation by caretakers in therapeutic procedures is an additional worthwhile objective. Reasonable kinds of activity are sought in support of speech training. Here the therapist assumes an important modeling function before the caretakers take on appropriate assignments (for example, monitoring and encouraging the program of self-modification). They are also involved in planned role playing. It is likely that simultaneous participation in therapeutic activities by several caretakers can provide a suitable training context as well as opportunity for them to address difficulties they have with each other.

Wendlandt (1972) suggests that group practice of caretakers and stutterers comprises a basic component of therapy and that stutterers be apprised of this necessary step right at beginning of therapy. In our opinion this is absolutely required in the treatment of children. We shall return to the problem of parent-child management in the next chapter.

Support of therapeutic measures by caretakers is indeed constructive but we must not overlook the point that this circle of individuals has its limits for implementation of social therapy in most cases. It is certainly reasonable in individual cases also to involve the employer or a colleague of the stutterer. However, this is rarely attainable. Hence, it is all the more necessary to plan training steps carefully and to play them out beforehand so that clients are enabled to assume the responsibility for "try-out in emergency situations" on their own.

Wendlandt (1972) offers an array of additional stimuli to improve the process of resocialization of stuttering children. In the literature cited in this book, among other sources, the reader can find suggestions that bear on therapeutic measures concerned with initiation and monitoring of changes in the restricted and broader living environment of the stutterer. The central intent of the recommendations is to find a way for the stutterer and nonstutterer to proceed together. Wendlandt sees possibilities in trying to arrange for stutterers and nonstutterers to live together under therapeutic control. Such a project, though not unconditionally committed to constant supervision, fosters integration with the social activities of the participants, for example, arrangement of joint leisure and occupational activities. If such an intensive kind of collaboration is not possible, Wendlandt offers another suggestion, which aims at resocialization in a somewhat less obligatory form, the collaboration of stutterers and nonstutterers in the framework of groups organized for leisure-time activities. Here, too, an important function devolves upon the therapist if he or she desires a lasting transfer of results from therapy. The client and therapist must give thought constantly to possibilities as to how the stutterer can find people who have the same interests and hobbies as himself or herself. Sharing activities of existing clubs and organizations is one such possibility; organizing a club for stutterers and nonstutterers on their own is another. The obligations of self-organized groups might, indeed, present a real chance for the stutterer to acquire new and unfamiliar modes of collective behavior. However, normally, such organized social bonding is not likely to encourage single contact sources. Over a period of time the obligations are likely to deemphasize the most important context for learning, creating involvements (and also countering undesirable ones) that enable one to gain friends who are continuously helpful in the face of acute problems. On the other hand, a form of self-help can also grow out of such a club or organization, as has been found in the area of addiction, where results leave the efforts of many experts far behind.

SUMMARY

Management of social behavior disorders of stutterers is all the more imperative the longer the speech disorder has persisted. Fixed behaviors manifested in avoidance of social contacts lead to substantial knowledge and competence gaps on the part of many clients. Treating speech disorders promises only poor results if it is not coordinated with basic training in the acquisition, broadening, and modification of social skills. Detailed recommendations to accomplish this have been given. The application of role playing as a medium of therapy and participation in therapy by caretakers were proposed as possibilities. Systematic implementation of social therapeutic measures was recommended. In the next chapter comprehensive structuring and implementation of complex programs of therapy will be detailed. Differentiated therapy for children, adolescents, and adults will be addressed.

Chapter 10

Combination of Speech and Social Therapeutic Measures in the Treatment of Stuttering

INTRODUCTION

In previous chapters distinctive aspects of treatment of stuttering were singled out and presented in detail. We have pointed out that the single measures that have been advanced do not by themselves do justice to the multifaceted nature of the conditions involved in stuttering. It is not without reason that in current practice there are increasing efforts to integrate differing therapeutic approaches into broader aspects of treatment. Consequently, we have formulated several requirements that need to be considered in combining individual methods in therapy.

(1) Above all the planned combination of methods needs to take into account individual determinants; included are

- present expression of the speech disorder and its contribution to constraint of overall oral motor activity
- ongoing self-perception and self-control of the stuttering on the part of the client
- situation-specific assessment of his or her own communication responsibility and communication competence (affective and cognitive-social determinants)
- availability as well as limitations of skills in social behavior.

(2) To satisfy the need for resocialization adequately social determinants have to be included. Relevant is pertinent information about the intimate living environment of the stutterer, about the lifestyles of family, friends, and colleagues, as well as about social demands on the stutterer, not to mention indifference to such demands. Distinctive aspects of specific situations need to be considered, especially those that have an effect

on responsibility for communication. Also included here would be conditions characterizing the broader life milieu, particularly the group-specific standards of social conduct (organizational, political, religious).

(3) We should make certain that the therapeutic procedures open the possibility for early dispensing with the therapist. This is the case even when the prognosis is not very favorable, as with cases of very severe disorder (Chapter 11). Continuation of treatment can be transferred to the client himself or herself (guidance of the client to self-modification). Client and caretakers can be assigned a common responsibility for continuing treatment (early involvement of key caretakers in therapy).

. (4) In this recapitulation we see once again that children and adults require different approaches. Among other reasons, this is necessitated by the varying stages in symptom development, by age-dependent capacity for self-control, and by distinctive complexity of social determinants.

In this chapter we shall subdivide our exposition of this last point. We shall deal first with early considerations and early treatment of childhood stuttering. Ideas on the formulation and implementation of therapy pro-. grams for adolescent and adult stutterers will follow. Finally, several current approaches involving a combination of methods will be presented and their claims evaluated.

EARLY IDENTIFICATION OF STUTTERING

The earliest possible identification of stuttering in children is generally considered to be a prerequisite for successful treatment (among others, Böhme, 1977; Ingham & Andrews, 1973a). A substantial number of spontaneous remissions has also been observed in children (Sheehan & Martyn, 1966). Obviously, the age of the stutterer and the length of time of the stuttering exert a considerable influence on the results of treatment and on the proportion of relapses.

Yet, time and again Johnson has made it clear that in early determination of disorder (mostly by caretakers) there is the danger that this is the original cause of stuttering (Chapter 3). In our model (Chapter 4) we referred to our agreement with his notion. Inherent in early identification and diagnosis is the problem of accentuating development of symptoms, especially where caretakers strive for a speedy elimination of difficulties by demanding more self-discipline of the child ("After all, try once again").

If parents seek an early consultation at the point in time of so-called developmental stuttering (the stage of normal disfluencies without situational variables), they should be informed of the course of normal speech development. It should be emphasized that disfluencies of speech are seen in all children. Parents should be counseled not to take notice of them while at the same time to affirm fluent and unruffled speech. Unruffled fluent speech clearly depends on situational factors. Parents should try to create circumstances where the child can speak smoothly, without pressure and without aggravated communication responsibility. Frequent communication with the child in a variety of situations can overcome deficits in verbal expression. In our opinion it is necessary to do this if we want to make available to the child ample opportunities in different situations to focus on the content of what is said (Widlak & Fiedler, 1977).

Several kinds of effective prophylaxes are commendable. In the long term, physicians, psychologists, and speech therapists should try to guide existing practices in order to prepare the parents for the tasks of rearing the child. Parents should receive more information about acquisition of language and speech and about prevention of speech disorders. This can be broadened effectively to include appropriate media (newspapers, periodicals, radio, and television).

EARLY TREATMENT OF CHILDHOOD STUTTERING

In the early development of the speech disturbance increasingly frequent interruptions in fluent speech as a reaction to situational demands or as a consequence of emotional-cognitive agitation are observed. If a child is seen in this phase then clarification of parent-child interaction is in order (Motsch, Affeld-Niemeyer, Bader, & Hoefert, 1977). Questions are asked as to whether frequent communicative and emotional conflicts appear and if these conditions of conflict affect the speech behavior of the child. Whether the child has shortcomings in tolerating situational pressure can be noted. The analysis of interaction sheds light on what circumstances precede disfluencies (for example, an expressed demand for fluent speech) and what events follow (for example, punishment for disfluencies). For clarification of the interacting modes of the child observation of behavior in his or her natural life context is preferable to observation of parent-child interaction in the therapy room (Shames & Egolf, 1976; Schulte & Kemmler, 1974). Systematic observation of this kind offers numerous points of departure for therapy.

When a child stutterer is brought to a therapist it is wise to reach an agreement committing the parent to participation in the therapy right from the start. Parents vary in their willingness to go along with such a request (it is indeed the child who stutters and needs treatment and not they). It has been our experience, nevertheless, that parents are ready to cooperate if they are made to believe that results will be achieved sooner if they support the efforts of the therapist (as cotherapists, so to speak). They are with the child almost the entire time between therapeutic sessions. Only they can ensure reasonable continuity of treatment.

If the observation of interaction indicates that parents exert excessive pressure on the child and make great demands on his or her speech behavior, then a high-priority goal of treatment is to eliminate the conditions that trigger stuttering. By observing the therapist as model the parent learns to contrive situations in which the child can speak fluently without demands to do so. Such situations should be as playful as possible. Puppet plays, dramatic presentations, guessing games, and "wars of words" are suitable media. They can be arranged so as to progressively increase requirements for the child to play along. It also helps here to ignore disfluencies and to affirm fluent speech and, above all, the content of what is said! Video recordings are useful in communicating appropriate model behavior to parents. Video recordings of parent-child interaction can enhance the learning effect of immediate practice. Recommendations on video feedback have been made in Chapters 7 and 9.

If the speech difficulties appear to be firmly fixed, then treatment takes the particular circumstances into account. Speech techniques for modifying a pattern of stuttering are not used in children under six years of age. Procedures are carried out in a way that the child's attention is diverted from disfluencies while talking. We have noted in the approach of Calavrezo that practice in talking with gestures is very effective in therapy (see also Chapter 6). The therapist can suggest gesture play in which children must use their hands, arms, or their whole body in exaggerated fashion in order to communicate ("as correctly as an actor") what they want to say, what they think, and what they experience and feel within themselves. Children seize upon this kind of play because it allows for activity that has heretofore been repressed (for example, the "flight" of a bird reported with outspread and swinging arms who informs "bird children" listening on the radio that in her flight she can observe everything that is going on in the playroom; or an illustrative description of an object not in the room and which the therapist must visualize correctly).

Occasions should be created in all play therapy that afford the child numerous opportunities to speak (suggestions can be found in Hilsheimer, 1975). Also the value of rhythmic and psychomotor training should not be overlooked. It has been shown that there is a relation between speech and motor activity. "Motor clumsiness" of many stuttering children has been universally reported (for example, Führing, Lettmayer, Elstner, & Lang, 1976). Schilling and Krüger (1959/60) have reported significant correlations between stuttering and various degrees of motor retardation. And Luchsinger (1948) has shown that progress in fine-motor ability is associated with improvement in speech and language disorders.

Psychomotor training has been used increasingly in children with cerebral disfunction. Where there is mild cerebral disfunction in stutterers along with fine-motor difficulties the introduction of rhythmic or psychomotor measures should be considered (Böhme, 1977).

Elsewhere we have called attention to the symptom-reducing effect of rhythmic speech (Chapter 6). Rhythmic exercises with the tambourine, clapper, and such are suitable for metronome training with children. Then the rhythm expressed in movement (for example, beating on the tambourine) is extended stepwise to speech. Allowance is made individually for differing levels of speech difficulty (whispering as well as loud and soft speech), which can be improved in steps. Speech anxieties may also be reduced in this way. Suitable, too, are clapping exercises with and without speech, which can then be combined with breath-controlled singing (examples can be found in Stange, 1970).

The use of pantomime and improvisation has been shown to be especially useful in rhythmic training. This requires silent expressive behavior. The gestures that have been worked out (comparable to the Calavrezo exercise, Chapter 6) are later accompanied by speech. Generally, these drills afford an abundance of opportunities to influence speech, self-confidence, and verbal expression positively. These exercises are also conducive to adequate social behavior, especially when they are performed in groups. In all of these procedures unnecessary emphasis on the disorder is avoided, since no prominence is given to the treatment of speech itself. Other practical exercises can be found in Hünnekens and Kiphard (1963), Zuckrigl and Helbling (1976), and Führing et al. (1976).

If these measures stabilize the speech then the parents are drawn in step by step. At first they observe the therapist-child interaction; then gradually they take over the role of therapists.

We point out once again that therapy exclusively for speech promises a result only if the factors that are jointly responsible for inducing stress have been eliminated and if the child has been guided to self-acceptance of his or her role as a talker. To help with this, additional therapeutic measures are available, especially role playing by which alternative modes of behavior are tried out and systematically used. Deidenbach (1977) reported a case of mother-child management in which he tried to resolve a conflict between mother and child using puppets. Even if a child who did not stutter was involved this would be useful as a systematic procedure.

First an observed interaction conflict between mother and child was recorded by the therapist (in the role of mother) and the assistant (in the role of child) using Punch and Judy puppets in varied problem situations.

Video and sound recordings were made. Then the therapist and assistant (in the same roles) presented a previously worked out resolution model of the same interaction with puppets. Again video and sound recordings were made. Both video recordings were played to the child with the request that he seek the best way out. Then the assistant (as mother) and the child freely recorded the scene again with puppets. The child chose a procedure similar to the one in the resolution model. Finally, the three video tapes were played to the mother one after another. Then she herself and the child freely recorded their role performance (likewise with puppets); both opted for the resolution model. The child was given cassettes containing all the sound records to take home with him. There, it was reported, he listened almost exclusively to the last sequence (the conflict resolution model with mother) and proudly played it for several friends and relatives. Following more such single sessions the interactive habits between mother and child were altered substantially.

We consider it vitally important that the parents encourage the child to do a good deal of talking. Thus, the child gets pleasure out of communicating. Furthermore, avoidance of conversational and situational behavior that can result in social difficulties is obviated.

THE TREATMENT OF STUTTERING IN OLDER CHILDREN AND YOUTHS

In this section we take up problems that are also relevant to the treatment of adult stutterers. In the four preceding chapters we described in detail singular methods applicable to them. Later sections dealing with efficient combinations of methods can be applied in principle to older children and youths. However, we need to keep in mind the particular characteristics of their stage of social development and the status of the speech disorder.

While we do not have to emphasize the speech disorder per se in treating stuttering in early childhood, maturation and especially increasing symptomatology raise the question of instituting a sequence of therapeutic steps. A second problem involves choice of method suitable for the age level. And third, a more significant question has to do with the positive transfer to everyday situations of what has been learned in therapy, the more so since with the advancing age of their children parents are less moved to cooperate and finally assume no responsibility as a cooperating participant in therapy of the youthful stutterer.

SEQUENCE OF THERAPEUTIC STEPS

With the growing complexity of the symptom picture stuttering affects the general behavior repertoire of the stutterer increasingly and more intensely. Limitations on motor communication produce retardation of social development, which, as we have noted, is reflected in the avoidance of social situations, which in turn intensifies social awkwardness (Chapter 9). The most sensible way to break up this frequently encountered complex of conditions (anxiety-avoidance-incompetence) is to give priority to the treatment of anxiety. This means a sequence of treatment that must be aimed at a reduction of the various components of anxiety, for example, expectancy of stuttering as a consequence of certain experiences in communication responsibility, fear of stuttering, fear of negative consequences of stuttering, frightening and oppressive experiences (during a seizure of stuttering) of feeling helpless and, despite all efforts, of being unable to do anything about it, etc. If the fear of social situations can be reduced and the consequent aggravated feeling of communication responsibility diminished, then we can expect the need for continuous auditory self-control of speech output to be reduced and the disfluencies to be decreased.

Preparatory Phase

The preparatory phase of therapy has a decided influence on subsequent therapeutic steps. It serves to establish and to structure expectancy attitudes and adjustments that should facilitate changes in behavior or at least make them possible. If these cognitive-social components are not taken into account, hardly any positive transfer will take place since an unaltered negative self-valuation results in increased stuttering due directly or indirectly to accentuated tendencies toward self-observation (i.e., auditory control of the stuttering). Here the crucial problem of the therapist is not so much to establish fluent speech but to maintain the awareness of one's own symptoms. The course for this is set in the preparatory phase. The following specific steps for implementation are suggested (Widlak & Fiedler, 1977):

- Removal of the taboo on stuttering (insofar as this is possible with children); this can happen by
- explanation of the neuropsychological conditions causing the symptoms; or by
- experiential training that illustrates the variation in speech difficulties under varying conditions of communication responsibility. For example,
- explanation of normal functioning of organs of speech (chewing, whistling, whispering, counting, speaking monosyllables, singing alone or in a chorus, etc.)

- immunization against disfluencies and the occasions of negative reactions to stuttering by listeners (by training in self-confidence through role playing, by practice in positive self-instruction, etc.).

Establishing Fluent Speech

In the second phase of therapy the vital question of establishing fluent speech is addressed. The problem has been adequately taken up in previous chapters. Here we only stress once again that every sort of aid to speech requires very careful planning in approaching normal speech. This applies especially to techniques of speech training that aim to develop a mode of talking leading to fluent speech, such as paced or prolongated speech.

Producing Conditions for Positive Transfer

The primary objective of the third phase is to reduce the responsibility of the therapist more and more and to transfer it to the client and/or his or her caretakers. Parents and other relevant caretakers are very important as cotherapists in the transfer and maintenance phase: They should be able to implement independently the techniques used by the therapist in the therapy situation. Negative situational influences and overtaxing conditions need to be eliminated. If this is not possible the child is prepared for aversive stimulations (his or her immunization). Talking, whether with or without failure, should be self-reinforcing, that is, it should be valued and experienced positively ("talking is easy!" "talking is fun!" "silence is no fun!" etc.). The speech techniques that have been initiated for avoidance of disfluencies are judged by the client to be less conspicuous than his or her original symptoms and are considered socially acceptable forms of communication. Otherwise positive transfer can hardly be expected.

Not only difficulties of communication but also problems in achievement can occur in the course of development of stuttering. These too must be tackled in therapy, as the following example makes clear: A thorough behavior analysis may reveal that various teachers react with great consideration to the stuttering of students. This is apparent when the student voluntarily announces that he or she hardly has anything to say, or at a given moment when he or she obviously cannot get out another word and refrains from answering a question. In this way the student shows his or her good intentions and simultaneously contrives to pass up the possibility of being compared with fellow students (negative reinforcement). (It should be emphasized explicitly that here the stutterer does not stutter intentionally.) We can presume strong motivation for learning if we assume that such students do their homework completely and carefully. It is more likely that the assigned homework will not be completed. However, this approaches a "gain from illness," which, while tolerated, results perhaps in increasingly larger gaps in knowledge. In the course of time the student "needs" his or her symptomatology to prevent the gaps in achievement from becoming well known. Similar strategies apply to many other behaviors, not just stuttering.

COMBINED METHODS

It is clear that the therapist must not pass up combining several different single procedures if his or her treatment is to do justice to the complexity of the disorder. We shall now present and briefly evaluate familiar combinations of methods. In addition to those references dealing with single methods mentioned in previous chapters, the cited methods will help the reader put together programs suited to individual situations.

MULTIDIMENSIONAL THERAPEUTIC APPROACHES

Recognizing the multifactored structure of the stuttering syndrome, Böhme (1977) recommends that designs for treatment be sought that are most in accord with individual findings and with the current state of knowledge. He himself proposes what he calls "multidimensional therapy." He distinguishes between *basic* and *differential* therapy to accommodate age-related differences among stuttering clients. The first step (the basic procedure) consists of systematic practice in new modes of speech behavior accomplished by the following single steps:

1. Preventative stopping: By timely interruption of speech the client learns to recognize and consequently to control the kinesthetic stimuli associated with the occurrence of stuttering symptoms.
2. Overall relaxation: This will be inserted after the stops in order to enable a relaxed new start toward speech fluency.
3. Breathing aids are introduced after the stops as supplementary measures for a more fluent start in speaking and for the desired relaxation.
4. Finally, other speech aids are included.

Böhme believes that the basic therapy can be systematically applied to preschool children but not later than to those of school age. It is used regularly in different conversational situations and after improvement in speech behavior is replaced by differential therapy directed to specific objectives.

This differential therapy takes into account to a much greater extent the distinctive characteristics of the stuttering syndrome in each individual case. Various measures are introduced simultaneously or are arranged sequentially. Decisions are primarily based on the age of the stutterer: At the preschool level, along with the treatment of speech, consultations with parents concerning training, systematic expansion of vocabulary of the stuttering child, other aids such as shadow speech following the so-called "unisono-method" of Liebmann (1914), or rhythmic speech are included. Böhme suggests indications for specific measures in individual cases. At the school-age level differential therapeutic procedures need to consider particularly the stress of school and the pressure to achieve. Hence, additional measures such as training in cognitive self-evaluation and self-instruction are indicated (following recommendations for behavior therapy of Meichenbaum, 1977), which stress improvement of self-control and self-assertion of child stutterers. Finally, for youths and adults the central focus of therapy is the improvement of interpersonal communication. Fears associated with talking are treated mainly by therapeutic behavioral methods and psychotherapeutic discussion. For all age levels Böhme gives advice for supplementing the procedures with pharmacological treatment.

Although we have reservations about the recommendation of medication, Böhme's other suggestions for treatment have advantages, not the least of which is planning for therapeutic objectives stated in terms of combining discrete requirements. This affords an overview in therapy for the entire scope of the symptom complex. The therapist is thus required to come to a goal-directed understanding of the manifold levels of the disorder (speaking, accessory symptoms, neurophysiological correlates, social determinants).

Seeman (1969) has developed another distinctive multidimensional therapeutic model that takes into account the manifold levels of determinants of stuttering. Changing social situations that give rise to conflict and elimination of fears of speech are prominent features of his method. Seeman's method employs psychotherapeutic intervention involving caretakers (primarily parents of stuttering children) preparatory to and during therapy. Explanation and information to parents about causes and the necessary conditions for changes in stuttering go along with the efforts of the therapist to eliminate speech fears of stutterers and to enable them to come to positive terms with their speech disorders. With this in mind training procedures are included in therapy that have as their aim alteration of breathing behavior, acquisition of relaxation techniques, learning a new manner of speaking by practice in reading and conversing, as well as attending to patterns of language. To center the stutterers' attention on other aspects of communication situations association exercises are employed in which the stutterers are urged to practice rapid construction of sentences or the use of complex word patterns systematically.

In our opinion Seeman's recommendations combining psychotherapeutics and instruction are appropriate, especially for children. As an intergral component of his "complex treatment" Seeman suggests drug support for "easing of stuttering and for elimination of dissonance in the somatic nervous system" (p. 343). In this connection we have repeatedly commented on the value of improving opportunities for externally and self-initiated procedures for relaxation to reduce the effects of general and specific agitating circumstances. This also applies to relaxation treatment for children (Hilsheimer, 1975).

Another widely known multidimensional concept is that of Fernau-Horn (1969), which attempts to apply individualized age-adapted therapy (to the stutterer) and social therapy (to interlocutors, chiefly to parents). A detailed differential diagnosis is carried out in each case with the aim of objectively informing ("enlightening") the stutterer as well as caretakers about the causes of stuttering and the therapeutic possibilities for change. Calming of speech behavior is achieved by breathing and relaxation techniques and "easing" of communication conditions is accomplished by social intervention. A wide variety of treatments is included to ensure transfer. They range from deliberate shaping of intent (autosuggestion) to therapeutic conversations including rhythmic and psychomotor practice.

INTEGRATIVE BEHAVIOR THERAPY FOR STUTTERING

As a consequence of a number of individual case studies we ourselves have attempted to combine different procedures for adult stutterers, especially in those aspects of our total program of treatment involving behavior therapy (Schmidt & Standop, 1974; Hofmann, Oertle, & Reincke, 1975; Fiedler, 1976). Our goal was to achieve meaningful integration of speech and social therapy in a manner that would make possible the gradual fading out of the therapist from therapeutic activities and would lead clients to beneficial continuation of therapy on their own (self-modification). It is clear from Figure 10-1 that this requires simultaneous operation on two therapeutic levels. Level I comprises systematic training in new modes of speaking and in social skills; Level II progressively familiarizes clients with strategies for self-control and self-modification, the use of which they should try out and establish firmly.

Figure 10-1 Summary of the Approach to Integration of Speech and Social Therapeutic Measures (Level I) as well as Acquisition and Implementation of Self-Modification (Level II)

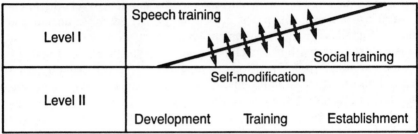

Speech Therapy on Level I

Our approach to speech training is similar to the basic therapy of Böhme. At first, clients are instructed in methods of perception of symptomatic and symptom-free speech in varying situations and under differing conditions. They are instructed simultaneously in methods of "progressive muscle relaxation" with special emphasis on the muscle groups participating in the speech act. Practice in easy breathing helps in relaxation training. These three training approaches are very soon combined to achieve controlled speech (first in therapy, then in situations outside of therapy). The procedures are individually tailored to each client. This means that when the client notes that he or she is disfluent (i.e., that attention is again focused on symptoms), then he or she should stop immediately ("stop!"). He or she redirects attention to his or her bodily state and tries to assume a relaxed state ("relax!"), and in so doing breathes in easily ("breathe!") and then finally begins to speak ("speak!"), continuing to concentrate as much as possible on the maintenance of relaxation.

Introduction of additional aids to speech is advisable if stuttering symptoms are severe. For this we have generally preferred paced speech using the metronome or haptometronome. However, with the use of additional combined aids to speech it is advisable to specify criteria in the course of therapy as to which method should be used under external conditons.

Social Therapy on Level I

After a few speech training sessions we begin social training, which in our therapy regularly involves a tripartite pattern comprising (1) "verbal structuring," (2) "role playing with feedback," and (3) "testing actions that address everyday demands."

To begin with, the client is requested to make himself or herself comfortable, to relax somewhat, and then to envisage designated problem levels from a hierarchy of social problem situations that had been drawn up previously. With the assistance of speech help as the situation may require, the client is asked to verbalize *loudly* the pertinent determinants of the problem, his or her own role in relation to the problem that has been selected, as well as possible actions aimed at its solution. The purpose of verbal structuring is to achieve a relaxed (i.e, desensitizing) cognitive analysis of past (or even future) circumstances associated with problems. In the search for problem-solving action the therapist must be prepared to lend a helping hand to the discussion especially if the client lacks inspiration.

As soon as possible after this, one or two role plays with video feedback are carried out in which the client attempts to test and to improve on problem-solving actions (we have described the actual procedure in Chapter 9). At the conclusion of such a segment of therapy client and therapist explore possibilities for early transfer of the practiced social behaviors to intervals between therapeutic sessions and then plan them accordingly.

The results of testing actions that address everyday demands are discussed in the next therapy session. The experiences are then applied to further social training.

Self-Modification on Level II

Guidance of the client of self-modification of his or her stuttering (speech as well as social behavior) is the most important concern of therapy. Closely dovetailed with one another are three steps, development, training, and establishment, which must be applied to speech and social therapeutic measures together.

Development in this overall framework is understood to mean mediation in small steps of knowledge and experience dealing with sensori-motor regulation of at-will relaxation and with respiratory characteristics of disfluent and fluent speech. Clients are guided to careful self-observation and experience in a variety of situations associated with fluent and disfluent speech in order that they may become familiar as directly as possible with conditions that cause or change stuttering. Client and therapist explore possibilities for establishing and maintaining conditions that foster self-controlled changes in symptoms.

In training, aids to speech involved in speech and social therapy and newly acquired social capabilities are backed up by supplemental self-control (cognitive) measures. These include systematic practice in self-instruction and in rules of behavior (Meichenbaum, 1977; Fiedler, 1978a). The focal point of establishment is the combination of new modes of speaking and social capabilities under everyday conditions. As early in therapy as possible free time should be provided in which successes and failures in the use of learned behaviors and cognitive strategies in social contexts are discussed, thereby affording feedback and evaluation. Opportunities and methods are sought to enable the client to deal independently with future failures (relapses) and to undertake changes in self-modification on his or her own. The possibility needs to be considered that there may be circumstances for which it would be helpful for the client to call on the services of an expert (therapist) once again.

Overall therapy concludes with planning for appropriate posttherapeutic care. At the least, meetings can be arranged at the invitation of the client or of the therapist that deal with posttherapeutic follow-up.

Our experience with this approach leads us to assume that the observed improvements in speech behavior are due to the effective change of the client's attitude toward his or her own speech difficulties. This is obviously more difficult to achieve with older clients (over 30) than with younger adults. They, more than likely, would have had several therapists previously. Improvements in speech behavior were also noticeable at the beginning of social training. Improvements have been significantly stabilized with the increasing willingness of the client to use acquired social skills in everyday situations. We definitely recommend that at the earliest possible time appropriate aids to speech be sought which the client judges to be a form of help suited to his or her own speech needs.

Here, we refer briefly to other combinations of methods that are oriented to broadly based behavior therapy: Perkins (1973a, b; also Perkins, Rudas, Johnson, Michael, & Curlee, 1974) has suggested a program of treatment in which delayed auditory feedback (DAF) of speech (Chapter 6) is prominently used as an aid to speech and is withdrawn gradually. Along with this, additional speech and breathing training, psychotherapeutic discussions, as well as approaches that contribute to changes in the social milieu of the stutterer are carried out. The method was used with 17 adult stutterers three sessions per week over a period of three to four months. Substantial success was reported in more than two-thirds of the clients. Follow-up measures a half year after therapy indicated that the results were retained in only about half of the clients (however, only about 30% of a control group that had speech therapy showed similar results).

Brutten (1969) and Brutten and Shoemaker (1969) used a combined method involving a sequence of systematic desensitization (in sensu, Chapter 7), negative practice (Chapter 6), and systematic desensitization (in vivo,

Chapter 7). However, they considered that this combination, which they termed "inhibition therapy," was partially effective and then only with clients exhibiting severe emotional distress.

A procedure that seeks chiefly to modify internal (affective and cognitive) determinants of stuttering is role therapy, suggested by Sheehan (1970d). His approach focuses on the self-observation and self-perception of one's own speech disorders and on their underlying anxieties and conflicts. The stutterer is systematically guided to come to terms with his or her anxieties and helplessness and to accept his or her role as a stutterer. He or she also makes them clear to the outside world and does not conceal them ("make your stuttering a public event!" p. 291). Group work and performance in public are desirable objectives and aspects of the approach shared by therapist and client. Aids to speech (for example, prolonged speech and negative practice) are also included in therapy as well as additional exercises in breathing and relaxation.

A comprehensive approach that seeks to do justice to the multifaceted complex of stuttering by integrating various procedures is contained in the monograph of Van Riper (1973). Four interlocking phases characterize the concept of therapy he recommends: (1) In the identification phase the stutterer is guided by self-observation and self-exploration through experiences and analysis to recognize dependence of normal speech and stuttering on internal as well as social factors. (2) In the desensitization phase the emphasis is on treatment of anxieties tailored to the stutterer's particular situation. (3) In the modification phase stuttering is changed by aids to speech (largely by delayed auditory feedback as well as prolonged and rhythmic speech) and social behaviors are altered by role playing and self-instruction/self-control. (4) In the stabilization phase fundamental steps are taken to initiate and consolidate positive transfer. Van Riper's integrative procedures merit our attention, especially because of his more than 40 years experience in stuttering therapy.

Finally, we mention another multistage approach in which Zopf and Motsch (1973) combine logopedic and behavior methods. They aim to achieve a systematic, effective transfer from therapy in stepwise fashion by (1) relaxation training, (2) symptom awareness, (3) speech training, (4) systematic desensitization, (5) generalization, and (6) careful follow-up.

RESOCIALIZATION AS A CONCERN OF BEHAVIOR THERAPY

In Chapter 7 we mentioned the efforts of Wendlandt (1972) to extend speech therapy with the purpose in mind of restoring the stutterer as completely as possible to his or her normal life situation. Wendlandt recommends a sequence of treatment stages that are linked one to the other all the way to extensive therapeutic follow-up: Stage I of his therapy comprises training in symptom perception and symptom control by which a new and objective attitude of the stutterer toward his or her speech difficulties is built up. There is a timely overlap with Stage II in which various aids to speech are systematically practiced, especially to facilitate surmounting of symptoms. Stage III aims to transfer the skills acquired with the help of speech aids to a dynamic-accentuated manner of speaking (in Richter's sense, 1967). After these preparatory steps, Stage IV is increasingly directed to the task of preparing and supporting transfer of the symptom-free manner of speaking to a variety of everyday situations. For this, a targeted reduction of existing social behavioral disturbances is sought by means of social training in therapy and by progressive testing of acquired social skills in real conflict and anxiety situations. As a part of therapy Stage V involves a test of permanence of results through therapeutic follow-up. Here the therapist is expected to help in initiating change processes involving the stutterer and nonstutterers. For this, caretakers and other nonstuttering persons participate in therapeutic and posttherapeutic activities (Chapter 9).

Wendlandt attributes reported failures in treatment (in all schools of therapy) to the fact that facilitation of integrative therapy is not guaranteed to take place sufficiently on its own. The prospects for successful resocialization are continuously diminished if it is more or less left to chance. Under such circumstances, with a long history of symptom development, resocialization becomes just about impossible.

THE FUNCTION OF DIALOGUE IN THE TREATMENT OF STUTTERING

In clinical supervision we have observed how difficult it is for young and inexperienced therapists to get a firm handle on the treatment of extremely severe stutterers. The severity of the client's stuttering often exceeds the expectations (and understanding) of the therapist. At first, therapists reveal themselves to be extremely helpless and, finally, often exhibit behaviors that the stutterer experiences independently in normal social relations; avoidance of eye contact with the stutterer, impatience, increased assistance such as completing sentences begun by the stutterer, increased talking. We therefore recommend that therapists who are treating stutterers for the first time try either to prepare and organize their first therapeutic session not by themselves but together with a colleague or to arrange for sound or video recordings of themselves in order to facilitate control of the therapeutic dialogue and behavior by subsequent viewing and listening. Both measures are intended to preclude consolidation of premature, uncontrolled, detrimental behaviors and habits of interaction with clients in therapy.

The extent to which the behavior of therapists influences therapeutic outcomes has, to our knowledge, hardly been studied. Hofmann, Oertle, and Reincke (1975) suggest that behavior of therapists exerts a substantial influence, especially in changing self-evaluation and self-control of clients. In their studies of individual cases they regularly provided for a change of therapists in order to minimize the influence of the therapist as much as possible and to determine unequivocally which methods (and not the influence of therapists) contributed to improvement of results. They ascertained that continuous private and social stress on the part of the therapist reflected the expectations of the client and (until the situation was corrected) mitigated significantly against the client's coming to terms with his or her own problems.

Westrich (1971, 1978) assigned an important function to the conduct of the therapist in treating stutterers. According to him, stuttering can be traced back to a situation characterized by fear of "saying anything specific or of feeling an urge to advocate [his or] her own personal views while the stutterer, [himself or] herself insecure, fears the consequences and reactions of the outside world" (1971, p. 27). He believes that it is essential for the therapist in discussion with his or her client to work for a change in the client's experiences and attitude toward his or her stuttering. Westrich claims that deep sympathetic understanding and personal rapport of the therapist with the stutterer is one of the most important and desirable objectives in therapy (1971, p. 74). In line with the concept of psychotherapeutic dialogue he considers the following criteria as particularly pertinent to effecting constructive changes in the stutterer (1971, p. 75):

- the extent of verbalization by the therapist of the substance of the emotional experiences of the subject
- the extent of trying, striving, reflecting, self-exertion of the therapist
- the extent of heartfelt sympathy, appreciation, and emotional warmth of the therapist

We also believe that the therapist who tries to meet these criteria can make deep-seated changes in the life experiences of the client by engaging in discussion. It appears to us that client-centered dialogue is a necessary supplement (even in a context of structured therapy) and especially advisable where (1) it is concerned with the exploration for those conditions that are responsible for individual causes and maintenance of the speech disorder and where (2) the client is trying on his or her own to find approaches for changing old living habits supported by therapeutic learning experience. Nevertheless, we do *not* share the views of Westrich (1971) that psychotherapeutic dialogue is the only precondition for enabling the stutterer to deal with his or her speech disorder or social demands (internally controlled) over the long term. This criticism also applies to an array of therapeutic approaches oriented to depth psychology (for example, Schneider, 1953) which claim that "major" psychotherapy is the exclusive road to success.

SUMMARY

In this chapter various possibilities were presented for combining speech and social therapeutic procedures in treatment. Several known multidimensional and integrative therapeutic concepts were put forward and assessed. Another focal point of our comments dealt with the distinctive treatment of childhood stuttering. Manifold possibilities in speech therapy for parent-child therapy were pointed out. Finally, the overall function of therapeutic dialogue was briefly commented on. As a framework for interaction in therapy, client-centered psychotherapeutic procedures based on dialogue were considered to be advisable to supplement speech and social therapy.

Chapter 11

Results of Therapy and Prognosis

INTRODUCTION

In conclusion, we shall address some unsolved problems in stuttering research. Despite steadily growing knowledge about the origins of stuttering it has not been possible in recent decades to increase the number of successful results of treatment. We are still finding a success rate similar to that previously reported by Nadoleczny (1926): Only about one-third of the clients were discharged as cured at the conclusion of treatment, another third showed improvement, and a third remained unaffected (Arnold, 1948; Fitz, 1961; Schilling, 1965; Seeman, 1969; Arnold, 1970b). If we look at investigations of the frequency of relapses (see below) then this breakdown is all the more discouraging. Once again to state the problem clearly, the overall reports of failures (except for only slight deviations) are apparently thought to result from differing therapeutic approaches and their contradictory theoretical arguments.

In this chapter we shall briefly touch upon completed research dealing with therapeutic outcomes and prognosis. We shall discuss problems that grow out of studies dealing with validation of prognostic judgments. Furthermore, we shall raise several questions about the reasons for success and failure and shall attempt answers.

MEASUREMENT OF OUTCOMES OF TREATMENT

Comparison of the efficacy of varying therapeutic interventions is difficult, if not thoroughly impossible, because of the lack of uniformity of outcome criteria. Therefore, problems that we encountered time and again in compiling the following sections will be dealt with beforehand.

Improvement in speech behavior is considered by most authors to be the most fundamental criterion of success in the treatment of stuttering.

Several others add to this, among other criteria, expansion of social competence, changes in attitude toward one's own problems, successful resocialization, etc. However, methods of evaluation of improvements in speech behavior are not at all uniform. Usually, they involve measurements of free speech dealing with a variety of subjects, reading from a standard text to no one, one, or several listeners in a thoroughly relaxed atmosphere. No doubt, reliability of the data within the framework of a given therapy is generally assured by holding constant the conditions under which measurements are repeated. However, what is mostly overlooked is the point that precise, fluent speech in a variety of situations (for example, speaking with affect or under conditions of reduced or aggravated communication responsibility) is an eminently proper outcome criterion because as much as anything it satisfies the demands of the client for a successful result of therapy.

Measurements of results are hardly ever based on the criteria of clients, although they really are the ones to judge the success or failure of their therapy (Eickels, Fiedler, & Schäuble, 1978). When self-appraisal by the client is elicited in order to give the therapist some clue to the attitude of the client toward his or her problem, what is most often overlooked is that the internal standard on which the client bases his or her appraisal can be shifted during therapy. Thus, in the course of successful treatment the client's standard may change to such a degree that residual speech difficulties are assessed more rigorously than before, resulting in a drastically increased probability of the risk of relapse.

Moreover, the continuing attempt to use "degree of severity" of the speech disorder as an indicator of the outcome of therapy is exceptionally precarious because it is beset with many problems of measurement. Generally, quantitative indicators (i.e., frequency and often the duration of symptoms per unit of time) constitute the standard of choice for measurement of the severity of disturbance. What is often overlooked is that the degree of difficulty in this sense is decidedly and directly bound up with other cognitive, affective, and social factors. In our opinion the view that a "mild" disturbance generally warrants a more favorable prognosis is no more tenable than that a "severe" disturbance suggests the same chance for success as a "mild" one. Now and then the view is advanced that "mild" forms of disturbance (i.e., negligible speech difficulties) are difficult or even impossible to overcome because attitudes toward symptoms or demands for change must be considered to be hardly or not at all modifiable.

Most investigations lack post-therapeutic study. The problem here is that investigators do not take it upon themselves to refer to features of outcomes in differential analysis and evaluation of approaches to therapy.

And if postinvestigations are carried out they most often take place very soon after treatment. We believe six months is too soon. At the least, the duration of treatment should be a yardstick for determining the point in time for katamnesis. Time and again relapses are observed years after therapy. To our knowledge conditions associated with very late relapse have not been studied.

Looking back to the statistical results of failures and successes (one-third cured, a third improved, a third unchanged), we can draw the conclusion only that outcome statistics would be even more unfavorable if the problems we have mentioned are taken into account. This is all the more to be suspected since, as a rule, failures are not publicized. We presume that very many studies are withheld because they do not satisfy statistical requirements. This is unfortunate, since careful studies of failures can yield pointers on optimizing therapeutic management.

Age of Clients

Schilling (1965) analyzed outcomes of therapy with respect to age. He studied 200 clients ranging from 3 to 49 years of age. He assessed the outcome of therapy to be "good" and "very good" in 34.5% of the clients, "improved" in 32%, and "unchanged" in 33.5%. Analysis of four groups subdivided according to age clearly revealed that children have the best chance for a successful result through therapy. In the 16 to 47 age group, the chances for success are rather less probable. Various other authors have confirmed that stuttering is more resistant to therapy in older adolescents and adults (Bryngelson, 1935; Fitz, 1961; Seeman, 1969; Kehrer & Stegat, 1968). However, this documentation is, perhaps, relative if we bear in mind that the rate of spontaneous remission in children is substantial. In a study of 8,000 elementary school children, Milisen and Johnson (1936) found that about 42% of stuttering children outgrow their disorder without therapeutic support (also Chapter 1).

The greatest prospects for successful outcomes are found in the treatment of preschool children (Chapter 10). As Johnson (1956b) has stated, conferences with parents in which information is given about speech development and the development of stuttering often suffice. Schilling (1965) held a similar view. However, his results were negligible in treatment of preschool children whose quantitative and qualitative symptomatology was firmly fixed. These children presumably are already much more intensely disturbed emotionally.

Sex of Clients

As we have seen, the number of successful results differs between males and females. Girls appear to have better prospects than boys (Arnold,

1970b). At the adult level this is reversed. Women have lesser prospects for success than men (Arnold, 1970b; Case, 1960). Schilling (1965) found universally poorer results with female children and adults but considering the small size of his sample he felt he could not make a valid statement about an age-related factor. It is difficult to find an explanation of the greater resistance of women to therapy. Social factors probably play a decisive role. As Ammons and Johnson (1944) have said, stuttering by men is more socially acceptable than by women. However, more thorough investigation is necessary to determine whether the higher rate of failure among women may be traced to differing behavior of caretakers toward males and females.

Duration and Frequency of Treatment

A possible explanation for the great danger of relapse of stutterers after the conclusion of therapy has been the suggestion that the pattern of new behavior has not been sufficiently stabilized. Aside from substantive and methodological aspects, the question here is whether and to what extent duration of treatment and frequency of therapeutic contact influence a favorable prognosis.

Precise statements about duration of treatment with adult stutterers are not easily come by. Treatment stretching over years is no exception. Wendlandt (1972) interviewed stutterers whose average length of treatment was 3.16 years (this number includes several who received follow-up therapy). Frequently, there are cases of individual treatments that extend over a period of 3 to 5 years. However, we can deduce from a variety of investigations that very long duration of therapy is *no* better guarantee of a successful outcome (Westrich, 1971, p. 96).

Heese (1967) discusses the advantages and disadvantages of limiting the time course of therapy. He indicates that we should keep in mind that comfortable contact with the therapist frequently reduces the cooperation of the client since he or she equates a successful result with the termination of therapy. We think this problem really ensues only when the therapist ignores measures for resocialization outside of therapy. The more steps that are taken to reintegrate stutterers into their everyday living environment the more they will be able to dispense with the therapist (as their only interlocutor) in solving their problems.

Is intensive treatment over a short period of time more effective than therapy that stretches out much more that a year? Wendlandt (1972) pleads for time-limited "intensive treatment" for adult stutterers, by which he means an overall duration of six months comprising three weekly sessions each lasting about one and one-half hours (p. 103). He continues treatment of one therapy session per week only if the "strength of new habits" of the adult with respect to stuttering shows signs of waning.

The results of Case (1960) argue against a beneficial effect of more frequent therapeutic sessions. He found no difference in outcomes among persons who had one or two or even more frequent sessions per week. In this instance the findings dealing with frequency of therapy are limited only to clients with clonic rather than tonic symptoms. Incidentally, Case had better results with clonic types when combined with his particular method of treatment involving predominantly negative practice (Chapter 6).

The rationale for more frequent sessions argues that difficulties that crop up in real life situations, in transfer of what has been learned in therapy, can be headed off early by the therapist. In our treatment, in which the frequency of therapeutic sessions was systematically varied, clients repeatedly told us they found long intervals (one week) to be rather uncomfortable since their successes as well as their failures could not be thoroughly discussed with the therapist (Schmidt & Standop, 1974). Furthermore, if the superiority with respect to improvement in speech behavior of more frequent sessions (one versus three sessions per week) could be neither definitely confirmed nor refuted it appears that continuous guidance of the client is absolutely necessary, especially at the beginning of therapy. With increasing success, time intervals between sessions should be constantly extended so that given a longer period of therapy they do not have to be terminated abruptly.

RELAPSE AND REPETITION OF THERAPEUTIC EXPERIENCE

The number of stutterers who seek treatment once again or repeatedly after termination of therapy is substantial. This is attested to by the questionnaire study of "Institute for Speech Disorders, Berlin" reported by Wendlandt (1972). As much as 96% of the respondents (stutterers) had previously been treated for their speech disorder, 73% at least twice, 39% at least three times, 16% at least four times, and 11% at least five times. According to self-evaluation by the clients, about half of the treatments (47%) showed no success; 4% of the cases felt they were even worse off. Lasting improvement was reported in only 7% of all treatments. In 85% of the cases posttherapeutic deterioration to previous levels set in after successful therapy. The clients felt that 77% of treatments appeared to be ineffective.

This poll made it additionally clear that single approaches, such as exclusive use of speech aids or concentration on psychotherapeutic, predominantly psychoanalytic dialogue, were hardly or slightly helpful.

CAUSES OF RELAPSE AND IMPLICATIONS FOR THERAPY

The numbers mentioned above document the high risk of relapse rather shockingly. In concluding this book we take occasion to inquire into the possible causes of these unfavorable prognoses and to draw conclusions about their implications for the therapeutic task. Since no reliable investigations are available, we resort only to speculation. To the reader is left the decision as to whether and to what extent he or she should agree with our arguments. We think that several of the implications we suggest, which we already have taken into account in our own therapeutic activities, are within the limits of present-day feasibility. Our main concern is to inspire the therapist to try them out and even to go beyond them.

Failure of Positive Transfer

Provision for therapeutic measures in the period after therapy is consistently assured in only a few approaches. It seems to us that therapy that concentrates solely on technical improvement in speech behavior or seeks success only by psychotherapeutic dialogue has as little chance of assuring positive transfer as does therapy aimed at enhancement of social competence without regard to speech difficulties. We need to keep firmly in mind that

- there is a formidable array of reliable speech aids that can improve the speech of stutterers (Chapters 6 and 7)
- behavior therapy, in particular, affords opportunities for systematic enhancement of the social competence of clients (Chapter 9)
- self-control and self-modification of speech and social problems employing appropriate procedures can be included in therapy (Chapter 8).

Long-term success of treatment depends on the extent to which the therapist is able to incorporate either successively or simultaneously all of the possibilities in therapy (several illustrations for this are given in Chapter 10). In previous chapters we have repeatedly argued for this because of the multifaceted conditions associated with stuttering.

There are still several other crucial points related to positive transfer. These involve the requirements of therapy (see also Sieland & Schäuble, 1976). We believe that failure of transfer occurs

- when the therapist does not work to motivate the client for transfer. It is wrong to assume that a client will really, and always, in crucial situations use what he or she has learned and mastered in therapy. A new pattern of behavior is much more difficult and riskier to apply in everyday situations than it is in the protective atmosphere of the therapy room. Therefore, in the course of treatment conditions must be created that enable the client to acquire a feeling of confidence beforehand (i.e., motivation) that it also works on the "outside" and/ or to learn from failures

- when the client gets no help in making a decision as to which behavior pattern to use, when and for what purpose to use it. He or she must learn to distinguish between situations that are appropriate and inappropriate for particular strategies. For example, it is advisable to make known that he or she is a "stutterer" and that he or she be given adequate time to talk in many, though not in all, conversational situations. Now and then it is indeed appropriate to be silent. On the other hand, there are situations in which the client must speak. The longer social difficulties persist the less likely it is that the ability to discriminate among such situations will be available to the client

- when the therapist does not persist in "thematizing" the transfer problem. In every therapeutic session the therapist should ask: "Are you really certain, [client], that you are actually carrying out your purposes as they were established in therapy? And how can we prepare you for so doing here and now in our therapy session?" A point should be made of failure. The client must also be prepared for it. Assurance of transfer is never a problem of only the latest therapeutic session. It can be attained only if improvement in new modes of behavior in natural circumstances is a constant object of attention in therapeutic sessions

- when the therapist leaves the client entirely alone in the process of reintegration into his or her social milieu. Successful resocialization requires targeted support growing out of clearly formulated questions. Therefore, it is advisable from the start and necessary to make a point continually of "lifestyle" (family and friends), of problems in the school or work place, and of the client's desire for change.

The following points are also related to the transfer problem. We consider them so important that we devote independent sections to them.

Relapsing Clients

The repeated search of stutterers for therapeutic help (mostly with other therapists) affords opportunities for a new beginning and presents problems associated with it. If he or she can establish a new emphasis the new therapist certainly has a good chance to stimulate the client to hopeful and active cooperation immediately. Results of the inquiry to stutterers to which we referred indicate that it is not inevitable that stutterers who have previously experienced several ineffective treatments must continue to remain unsuccessful. However, we must keep in mind that negative therapeutic experiences, especially with several former therapists, can be additive. The therapist should always work up the positive and negative experiences of the client with his or her predecessors. These may reoccur, especially with respect to the client's expectations, from the new therapy. One of the major concerns at the state of the new therapy is to head off negative experiences and to restructure them. Much more so than with a client undergoing therapy for the first time, these current expectations, goals, apprehensions, and already "distorted" hopes need to be discussed openly. On the other hand, little or no time should be spent on expectations of failure, that is, therapy should bypass the existing "chasm of despair." This is a basis for finding a new beginning jointly. Now and then the therapist must raise his or her expectations above what may be the more modest ones of the client.

The Cure Mythology

Many therapists give clients the impression at the beginning of therapy that "stuttering" is not a very great problem, that somehow or other it can readily be worked out, and that if the client makes the effort and attends carefully to every step along the way a cure will follow. (Note the title and parts of the recent book by Schwartz, 1977). Without realizing that they have done so they often make claims for cure that they are not able to satisfy later. What do we mean by a "cure?" Somewhat fluent speech? Or even assurance of no relapse?

The reports of results presented in this chapter point to a rather pessimistic outlook, namely, that given the present state of therapeutic knowledge and skill a preponderant proportion of stutterers (adults) can barely hope for a lasting improvement in their speech behavior. Concealing this and suggesting prospects for cure that cannot be realized are among the most significant reasons for the failure of a great deal of therapy.

We recommend explaining comprehensively and factually to adolescent and adult clients not only the origins and conditions necessary for change but also by explanation enable them to make a realistic appraisal of the outcomes of treatment. What is meant here above all is a most far-reaching openness of therapeutic management. This also has the important aim of scaling down overly optimistic and, hence, unrealizable expectations of the client. Among other things this means

- the client should understand that complete freedom from symptoms through therapy is achieved only with a great deal of difficulty
- the client must constantly count on the probability that in some situations improvements in speech behavior can regress and, indeed, he or she must expect that there may be circumstances where his or her speech can be much worse
- therapy cannot guarantee a cure. But it can enable the stutterer to find a new approach to his or her problems and to acquire new modes of active, affective, and cognitive interaction with residual speech difficulties
- the old behaviors that are intertwined with the stuttering simply cannot be extinguished today or tomorrow. They have been around for a long time and can only be unlearned slowly. Traces remain that can break out again. On the other hand, such small success as is achieved fosters hope that improvements can subsequently be initiated and achieved again
- since there is a risk of relapse, the stutterer also needs to learn to live with his or her stuttering. To do this requires modes of behavior that enable the stutterer despite speech difficulties to meet social demands and to respond extensively to his or her own social desires. One must be prepared for relapse and other social difficulties by acquisition of other skills in self-modification. Criteria are needed as to when it is desirable to seek support of a therapist again
- finally, in cases where his or her own treatment has reached a limit the therapist needs to seek the help of qualified colleagues.

We are convinced that given the present-day state of the potential of therapy, it is sufficient simply to make modest claims that can be fulfilled realistically. We believe with Watzlawick (1977) that this point of view counters most effectively the illusion of complete success as well as the despair of total failure.

References

Adams, M.R., Moore, W.H.: The effects of auditory masking on the anxiety level, frequency of disfluency, and selected vocal characteristics of stutterers. J. Speech Hear. Res. 15 (1972), 572–578.

Adams, M.R., Popelka, G.: The influence of »time-out« on stutterers and their disfluency. Behav. Ther. 2 (1971), 334–339.

Ammons, R., Johnson, W.: Studies in the psychology of stuttering: XVIII. The construction and application of a test of attitude toward stuttering. J. Speech Dis. 9 (1944), 39–49.

Andrews, G., Harris, M.: The syndrome of stuttering. Heinemann, London 1964.

Angermeier, W.F.: Kontrolle des Verhaltens. Springer, Berlin 1972.

Angermeier, W.F., Peters, M.: Bedingte Reaktionen. Springer, Berlin 1973.

Arnold, G.E.: Die traumatischen und konstitutionellen Störungen der Stimme und Sprache. Urban & Schwarzenberg, Wien 1948.

Arnold, G.E.: Das Poltern: Tachyphemie. In: Luchsinger, R., Arnold, G.E. (Hrsg.): Handbuch der Stimm- und Sprachheilkunde, Band II., 3. Aufl. Springer, Wien 1970 (a), S. 525–554.

Arnold, G.E.: Die soziale Neurose des Stotterns: Dysphemie. In: Luchsinger, R., Arnold, G.E. (Hrsg.): Handbuch der Stimm- und Sprachheilkunde, Band II, 3. Aufl, Springer, Wien 1970 (b), S. 749–803.

Aron, M.L.: Nature and incidence of stuttering among a Bantu group of school going children. J. Speech Hear. Dis. 27 (1962), 116–128.

Azrin, N.H., Jones. R.J., Flye, B.: A synchronization effect and its application to stuttering by a portable apparatus. J. Appl. Behav. Anal. 1 (1968), 283–295.

Azrin, N.H., Nunn, R.G.: Habit-reversal: A method of eliminating nervous habits and tics. Behav. Res. Ther. 11 (1973), 619–628.

Azrin, N.H., Nunn, R.G.: A rapid method of eliminating stuttering by a regulated breathing approach. Behav. Res. Ther. 12 (1974), 279–286.

Bachrach, D.L.: Sex differences in reaction to delayed auditory feedback. Perceptual Motor Skills 19 (1964), 81–82.

Bacon, F.: Sylva sylvarum, or a natural history in ten centuries. Cent 4 (1627), 386.

Barbara, D.A.: Stuttering—a psychodynamic approach to its understanding and treatment. Julian, New York 1954.

189

Barber, V.A.: Rhythm as a distraction in stuttering. J. Speech Dis. 5 (1940), 29–42.

Becker, K.P.: Die logopädische Behandlung des Stotterns im System des Sprachheilwesens. Die Sonderschule, Beiheft 1, 1970.

Beech, H.R., Fransella, F.: Research and experiment in stuttering. 2nd Ed. Pergamon, New York 1971.

Bekesy, G.V.: Zur Theorie des Hörens bei Schallaufnahme durch Knochenleitung. Ann. Phys. 13 (1932), 111–136.

Berendes, J., Schilling, A.: Stimm- und Sprachstörungen. Schallplatte mit Leitfaden. Lehmanns, München 1962.

Berger, M.M. (Ed.): Videotape techniques in psychiatric training and treatment. Brunner/ Mazel, New York 1970.

Berman, P.A. Brady, J.P.: Miniaturized metronomes in the treatment of stuttering: A survey of clinicians' experience. J. Behav. Ther. exp. Psychiat. 4 (1973), 117–119.

Berry, M.F.: Developmental history of stuttering children. J. Pediat. 12 (1938), 209–217.

Biggs, B.E., Sheehan, J.G.: Punishment or distraction? Operant stuttering revisited. J. abnorm. Psychol. 74 (1969), 256–262.

Birbaumer, N.: Physiologische Psychologie. Springer, Berlin 1975.

Black, J.W.: The effect of delayed sidetone upon vocal rate and intensity. J. Speech Hear. Dis. 16 (1951) 56–60.

Blankenheim, H.: Möglichkeiten einer gezielten Stotterertherapie im Sprachlabor. Z. Heilpäd. 2 (1973), 118–120.

Bloodstein, O.: Conditions under which stuttering is reduced or absent. J. Speech Hear. Dis. 14 (1949), 295–302.

Bloodstein, O.: Stuttering as an anticipatory struggle reaction. In: Eisenson, J. (Ed.): Stuttering—A symposium. Harper, New York 1958, S. 1–69.

Bloodstein, O.: The development of stuttering: I. Changes in nine basic features. J. Speech Hear. Dis. 25 (1960a), 219–237.

Bloodstein, O.: The development of stuttering: II. Development phases. J. Speech Hear. Dis. 25 (1960b), 366–376.

Bloodstein, O.: The development of stuttering: III. Theoretical and clinical implications. J. Speech Hear. Dis. 26 (1961), 67–81.

Bloodstein, O.: A handbook of stuttering. National Easter Seal Society, Chicago 1969.

Bluemel, C.S.: Stammering and allied disorders. Macmillan, New York 1935.

Böhme, G.: Störungen der Sprache, der Stimme und des Gehörs durch frühkindl. Hirnschädigungen, Fischer, Jena 1966.

Böhme, G.: Das Stotter-Syndrom. Huber, Bern 1977.

Böhme, G., Botzer, R.: Minimale zerebrale Dysfunktion und Sprachstörungen. München. med. Wschr. 117 (1975), 1883–1886.

Boudreau, L.A., Jeffrey, C.J.: Stuttering treated by desensitization. J. Behav. Ther. exp. Psychiat. 4 (1973) 209–212.

Brady, J.P.: Metronome-conditioned speech retraining for stuttering. Behav. Ther. 2 (1971), 129–150.

Brady, J.P.: Metronome-conditioned relaxation: A new behavioural procedure. Brit. J. Psychiat. 122 (1973) 729–730.

Brady, J.P., Brady Ch. A.: Behavior Therapy of Stuttering. Folia phoniat. 24 (1972), 355–359.

Branch, C., Milner, B., Rasmussen T.: Intercarotic Sodium Amytol for the lateralization of cerebral speech dominance. J. Neurosurg. 21 (1964), 399–405.

Brandon, S., Harris, M.: Stammering—An experimental treatment programme using syllable-timed speech. Brit. J. Dis. Comm. 2 (1967), 64–68.

Brankel, O.: Fehlatmung bei Sprechstörungen, im besonderen bei Stottern. Die Sprachheilarbeit 3 (1959), 65–74.

Brown, S.F.: The loci of stuttering in the speech sequence. J. Speech Dis. 10 (1945), 181–192.

Browning, R.M.: Behavior therapy for stuttering in a schizophrenic child. Behav. Res. Ther. 5 (1967), 27–35.

Brutten, E.J.: Stuttering: Reflections on a two-factor approach to behavior modification. In: Gray, B.B., England, G. (Eds.): Stuttering and the conditioning therapies. The Monterey Institute für Speech and Hearing, Monterey 1969, pp. 81–89.

Brutten, E.J., Gray B.B.: Effect of word cue removal on adaption and adjacency: A clinical paradigm. J. Speech Hear. Dis. 26 (1961), 385–389.

Brutten, E.J., Shoemaker, D.J.: The modification of stuttering. Prentice-Hall, Englewood Cliffs, N.J. 1967.

Brutten, E.J., Shoemaker, D.J.: Stuttering: The disintegration of speech due to conditioned negative emotion. In: Gray, B.B., England, G. (Eds.): Stuttering and the conditioning therapies. The Monterey Institute for Speech and Hearing, Monterey 1969, pp. 57–67.

Bryngelson, B.: Sideness as an etiological factor in stuttering. J. genet. Psychol. 48 (1935), 204–217.

Bryngelson, B., Rutherford, B.: A comparative study of laterality of stutterers and non-stutterers. J. Speech Dis. 2 (1937), 15–16.

Burke, B.D.: Reduced auditory feedback and stuttering. Behav. Res. Ther. 7 (1969), 303–308.

Buscaglia, L.F.: An experimental study of the Sarbin-Hardyk Test as indices of role perception for adolescent stutterers. Speech Monogr. 30 (1963) 243 (abstract).

Buxton, L.F.: An investigation of sex and age differences in speech behavior under delayed auditory feedback. Diss., Ohio State University 1969. Zitiert nach Van Riper (1971).

Calavrezo, C.: Die Behandlung des Stotterns durch die Sprachgebärden. De Therapia Vocis et Loquelae I (1965), 399–401.

Calavrezo, C.: Video-Aufzeichnungen; Therapiedemonstrationen; persönliche Mitteilungen. Münster 1973.

Case, H.W.: Therapeutic methods in stuttering and speech blocking. In: Eysenck, H.J. (Ed.): Behaviour therapy and the neuroses. Pergamon, Oxford 1960, pp. 207–220.

Chase, R.A., Sutton, S., First, D., Zubin, J.: A developmental study of changes in behavior under delayed auditory feedback. J. genet. Psychol. 96 (1961), 101–112.

Cherry, E.C., Sayers, B.M.: Experiments upon the total inhibition of stammering by external control, and some clinical results. J. psychosom. Res. 1 (1956), 233–246.

Cherry, E.C., Sayers, B.M., Marland, P.: Some experiments on the total suppression of stammering; and a report on some clinical trials. Bull. Brit. psychol. Soc. 30 (1956), 43–44.

Coën, R.: Pathologie und Therapie der Sprachanomalien für Ärzte und Studierende. Wien 1886.

Coriat, J.H.: The nature and analytic treatment of stuttering. Proceedings of the American Speech Correction Association 1 (1931), 151–156.

Curlee, R.F., Perkins, W.H.: Effectiveness of a DAF conditioning program for adolescent and adult stutterers. Behav. Res. Ther. 11 (1973), 395–401.

Curry, F.K.W., Gregory. H.H.: The performance of stutterers on dichotic listening task to reflect cerebral dominance. J. Speech Hear. Res. 12 (1969), 73–82.

Daniels, E.M.: An analysis of the relation between handedness and stuttering with special reference to the Orton-Travis theory of cerebral dominance. J. Speech Dis. 5 (1940), 309–326.

Deidenbach, H.: Video-Mitschnitt einer Eltern-Kind-Therapie; persönliche Mitteilungen. Wiesbaden 1977.

Dickson, S.: Incipient stuttering and spontaneous remission of stuttered speech. Paper, read before annual meeting of Amer. Speech Hear. Ass. 1969. Zitiert nach Van Riper (1971).

Dieffenbach, J.: Die Heilung des Stotterns durch eine neue chirurgische Operation. Förster, Berlin 1841.

Djupesland, G.: Middle ear muscle reflexes elicit by acoustic and non-acoustic stimulation. Acta Oto-Laryngal. 188 (1964), 287–292. Zitiert nach Widlak (1977).

Djupesland, G.: Electromyography of the tympanic muscles in man. Intern. Audiol. 4 (1965), 34–41. Zitiert nach Widlak (1977).

Dollard, J., Miller, N.E.: Personality and Psychotherapy. McGraw-Hill, New York 1950.

Dostálová, J.F.: Elemente des autogenen Trainings in der Komplextherapie des Stotterns. Folia Phoniat. 26 (1974), 181–182.

Doubek, F., Pakesch, E.: Die zentralen kindlichen Sprechstörungen als diagnostisches und therapeutisches Problem. Wien. Klin. Wschr. 69 (1957), 781–787.

Douglas, E., Quarrington, B.: The differentiation of interiorized and exteriorized stuttering. J. Speech Hear. Dis. 17 (1952), 377–385.

Downton, W.: The effect of instructions concerning mode of stuttering on the breathing of stutterers. In: Johnson, W. (Ed.): Stuttering in children and adults. 2nd Ed. Univ. of Minnesota Press, Minneapolis 1956, pp. 282–285.

Dührssen, A.: Psychogene Erkrankungen bei Kindern und Jugendlichen. Göttingen 1971.

Dunlap, K.: The technique of negative practice. Amer. J. Psychol. 55 (1942), 270–273.

Egolf. D.B., Shames, G.H., Blind, J.J.: The combined use of operant procedures and theoretical concepts in the treatment of an adult female stutterer. J. Speech Hear. Dis. 36 (1971), 414–421.

Egolf, D.B., Shames, G.H., Seltzer, H.: The effects of time-out of stutterers in group therapy. J. Comm. Dis. 4 (1971), 111–118.

Eickels, N.V., Fiedler, P. A., Schäuble, W.: Verhaltensmodifikation und Aktionsforschung. In: Fiedler, P.A., Hörmann, G. (Hrsg.): Aktionsforschung in Psychologie und Pädagogik. Steinkopff, Darmstadt 1978, S. 55–68.

Eisenson, J.: Observation of the incidence of stuttering in a special culture. J. Amer. Speech Hear. Ass. 8 (1966), 391–394.

Eisler, R.M., Hersen, M., Miller, P.M.: Effects of modeling on components of assertive behavior. Behav. Ther. Exp. Psychiat. 4 (1973), 1–6.

References   193

Fairbanks, G.: Systematic research in experimental phonetics: 1. A theory of speech mechanism as servosystem. J. Speech Hear. Dis. 19 (1954), 133–139.

Fenichel, O.: The psychoanalytic theory of neurosis. Norton, New York 1945.

Fernau-Horn, H.: Die Sprechneurosen. Hyppokrates, Stuttgart 1969.

Fiedler, P.A.: Gesprächsführung bei verhaltenstherapeutischen Explorationen. In: Schulte, D. (Hrsg.): Diagnostik in der Verhaltenstherapie. Urban & Schwarzenberg, München 1974, S. 128–151.

Fiedler, P.A.: Zur Funktion der Verstärkung in Problemlösungsprozessen. Phil. Diss., Münster 1975.

Fiedler, P.A.: Probleme in der Therapie eines erwachsenen Stotternden mit seltener Symptomatik. In: Reiss, M., Fiedler, P.A., Krause, R., Zimmer, D. (Hrsg.): Verhaltenstherapie in der Praxis. Kohlhammer, Stuttgart 1976, S. 63–71.

Fiedler, P.A.: Diagnostische und therapeutische Verwertbarkeit kognitiver Verhaltensdeterminanten. Praktische Ansätze für eine kognitive Verhaltenstherapie. In: Hoffmann, N. (Hrsg.): Grundlagen kognitiver Therapien. Huber, Bern 1978 (a).

Fiedler, P.A.: Zur Theorie und Praxis verhaltenstherapeutischer Gruppen. In: Die Psychologie des 20. Jahrhunderts, Band VII: Lewin und die Folgen, hrsgg. von A. Heigl-Evers, U. Streek. Kindler, München 1978 (b).

Fiedler, P.A., Hörmann, G. (Hrsg.): Aktionsforschung in Psychologie und Pädagogik. Steinkopff, Darmstadt 1978.

Fierman, E.Y.: The role of cues in stuttering adaptation. In: Johnson, W. (Ed.): Stuttering in children and adults. 2nd Ed. Univ. of Minnesota Press, Minneapolis 1956, pp. 256–263.

Fineberg-Garber, S., Martin, R.R.: The effects of white noise on the frequency of stuttering. J. Speech Hear. Res. 17 (1974), 73–79.

Fitz, O.: Schach dem Stottern. Freiburg i. Br. 1961.

Flanagan, B., Goldiamond, I., Azrin, N.: Operant stuttering: The control of stuttering behaviour through response-contingent consequences. In: Eysenck, H.J. (Ed.): Experiments in Behaviour Therapy. Pergamon Oxford 1964, pp. 173–177.

Florin, I.: Die Praxis der Systematischen Desensibilisierung. In: Florin, I., Tunner, W. (Hrsg.): Therapie der Angst. Urban & Schwarzenberg, München 1975, S. 241–267.

Florin, I., Tunner, W. (Hrsg.): Therapie der Angst: Systematische Desensibilisierung. Urban & Schwarzenberg. München 1975.

Flowers, J.V.: Simulation und Rollenspiel. In: Kanfer, F.H., Goldstein, A.P. (Hrsg.): Möglichkeiten der Verhaltensänderung. Urban & Schwarzenberg, München 1977, S. 178–219.

Foppa, K.: Lernen, Gedächtnis, Verhalten. Kiepenheuer & Witsch, Köln 1965.

Frank, A., Bloodstein, O.: Frequency of stuttering following repeated unison readings. J. Speech Hear. Res. 14 (1971), 519–524.

Frankl, V.E. Paradoxical Intention. Amer. J. Psychother. 14 (1960), 520.

Fransella, F., Beech, H.R.: An experimental analysis of the effect of rhythm on the speech of stutterers. Behav. Res. Ther. 3 (1965), 195–201.

Frasier, J.: An exploration of stutterers' theories of their own stuttering. In: Johnson, W. (Ed.): Stuttering in children and adults. University of Minnesota Press, Minneapolis 1956, pp. 325–334.

Freund, H.: Zur Frage der Beziehung zwischen Stottern und Poltern. Mschr. Ohrenheilk. 68 (1934), 1446–1457.

Freund, H.: Über inneres Stottern. Mschr. Ohrenheilk. 69 (1935), 146–148.

Freund, H.: Studies in the interrelationship between stuttering and cluttering. Folia phoniat. 4 (1952), 146–168.

Friedman, P.H.: The effects of modeling and role-playing on assertive behavior. In: Rubin, R.D., Fensterheim, H., Lazarus, A., Franks, C.M. (Eds.): Advances in behavior therapy. Academic Press, New York 1971, pp. 149–169.

Froeschels, E.: Eine Methode zur Behandlung von Sprechfurcht (»Stottern«, Assoziative Aphasie). Klin. Wschr. 3 (1924), 526–545.

Froeschels, E.: Twentieth century speech and voice correction. Philosophical Library, New York 1948.

Froeschels, E.: The significance of symptomatology for the understanding of the essence of stuttering. Folia phoniat. 4 (1952), 217–230.

Froeschels, E.: Selected Papers (1940–1964). North-Holland, Amsterdam 1964.

Früh, K.F.: Kybernetik der Stimmgebung und des Stotterns. Rentsch, Zürich 1965.

Führing, M., Lettmayer, O., Elstner, W., Lang, H.: Die Sprachfehler des Kindes und ihre Beseitigung. 6. Aufl. Bundesverl. f. Unterr., Wissensch. und Kunst, Wien 1976.

Gens, G.W.: The speech pathologist looks at mentally deficient child. Train. School Bull. 48 (1951), 19–27.

Glauber, I.P.: The psychoanalysis of stuttering. In: Eisenson, J. (Ed.): Stuttering: A symposium. Harper, New York 1958, pp. 71–119.

Goldiamond, I.: Stuttering and fluency as manipulatable operant response classes. In: Krasner, L., Ullman, L.P. (Eds.): Research in behaviour modification. Holt, New York 1965.

Goldman, R.: The effects of cultural patterns on sex ratio in stuttering. J. Amer. Speech Hear. Assoc. (abstract) 7 (1965), 370–371.

Goldman, R.: Cultural influence on the sex ratio in the incidence of stuttering. Amer. Anthrop. 69 (1967), 78–81.

Golub, A.: The cumulative effect of constant and varying reading material on stuttering adaptation. In: Johnson, W. (Ed.): Stuttering in children and adults. 2nd Ed. Univ. of Minnesota Press, Minneapolis 1956, pp. 237–244.

Graf, O.I.: Incidence of stuttering among twins. In: Johnson, W. (Ed.): Stuttering in children and adults. 2nd Ed. Univ. of Minnesota Press. Minneapolis 1956, pp. 381–386.

Graumann, C.F.: Motivation. Einführung in die Psychologie, Band 1. Huber, Bern 1969.

Grawe, K.: Verhaltenstherapeutische Gruppentherapie. In: Handbuch der Psychologie, Band 8. Klinische Psychologie, 2. Halbband hrsgg. von L. Pongratz. Hogrefe, Göttingen 1978.

Gregory, H.H.: Applications of learning theory concepts in the management of stuttering. In: Gregory, H.H. (Ed.): Learning theory and stuttering therapy. Northwestern Univ. Press, Evanston 1968, pp. 107–128.

Griffiths, R.D.: Videotape feedback as a therapeutic technique: Retrospect and prospect. Behav. Res. Ther. 12 (1974), 1–8.

Gumpertz, F.: Moderne Betrachtungsweisen zum Stotterproblem. Die Sprachheilarbeit 6 (1961), 1–7.

Gutzmann, A.: Das Stottern und seine gründliche Beseitigung durch ein methodisch geordnetes und praktisch erprobtes Verfahren. Berlin 1879.

Gutzmann, H. (sen.): Das Stottern. Eine Monographie für Ärzte, Pädagogen und Behörden. Rosenheim, Frankfurt/M 1898.

Gutzmann, H. (sen.): Sprachheilkunde, 2. Aufl. Kornfeld, Berlin 1912.

Gutzmann, H. (sen.): Übungsbuch für Stotternde, 19. Aufl. Neu hrsgg. von H. Gutzmann (jun.) und M. Nadoleszny. Osterwieck am Harz 1926.

Gutzmann, H. (jun.): Übung und Gewöhnung bei der Behandlung von Sprechstörungen (bes. Stottern). Med. Welt (1927), 46.

Gutzmann, H. (jun.): Gutzmanns Sprechübungsbuch. 23 Aufl. Hannover 1966.

Hamre, C.E., Wingate, M.E.: Pyknolepsy and stuttering. Quart. J. Speech 8 (1967), 374–377.

Haroldson, S.K., Martin, R.R., Starr, C.D.: Time-out as a punishment for stuttering. J. Speech Hear. Res. 11 (1963), 560–566.

Harris, W.E.: Studies in the psychology of stuttering XVII. A study of the transfer of adaptation effect in stuttering. J. Speech Dis. 7 (1942), 209–221.

Hartig. M. (Hrsg.): Selbstkontrolle. Urban & Schwarzenberg, München 1974.

Hartlieb, K.: Praktikum der Stimm- und Sprachheikunde. München—Basel 1969.

Haywood, H.C.: Differential effects of delayed auditory feedback on palmar sweating, heart rate, and pulse pressure. J. Speech Hear. Res. 6 (1963), 181–186.

Heese, G.: Zur Verhütung und Behandlung des Stotterns. Heilpäd. Beitr.: Schriften zur Pädagogik und Psychologie entwicklungsgehemmter Kinder, Heft 2. 3. Aufl. Berlin 1967.

Hennig, W.: Beiträge zur Erforschung des Stotterns und zum Aufbau einer Sprachgestörten-Fürsorge. In: Erziehung und Psychologie. Beiheft 12 der Zeitschr.»Schule und Psychologie«, München 1959.

Herscovitch, A., LeBow, M.D.: Imaginal pacing in the treatment of stuttering. J. Behav. Ther. exp. Psychiat. 4 (1973), 357–360.

Hilsheimer, G.V.: Verhaltensgestörte Kinder und Jugendliche, Maier, Ravensburg 1975.

Hoepfner, Th., Meyer, F.: Die Verhütung des Stotterns. Merkbuch für Lehrer und Erzieher. Wandsbek 1926.

Hofmann, H.J., Oertle, H., Reincke, R.: Überblick über die Stotterforschung und handlungstheoretische Perspektiven in bezug auf Einübung von Selbstregulation des Sprach- und Sozialverhaltens erwachsener Slotternder. Band I und II. Unveröff. Diplomarbeit, Münster 1975.

Holland, J.G., Skinner, B.F.: Analyse des Verhaltens. Urban & Schwarzenberg, München 1971.

Holliday, A.R.: The effect of meprobamate on stuttering. Fed. Proc. 18 (1959), 403.

Hull, C.L.: Principles of behavior. Appleton, New York 1943.

Hünnekens, H., Kiphard, E.: Bewegung heilt. Pschomotorische Übungsbehandlung bei entwicklungsrückständigen Kindern, 2. Aufl. Flöttmann, Gütersloh 1963.

Ingham, R.J., Andrews, G.: Behavior therapy and stuttering: A review. J. Speech Hear. Dis. 38 (1973 a), 405–441.

Ingham, R.H., Andrews, G.: An analysis of a token economy in stuttering therapy. J. Appl. Behav. Anal. 6 (1973b), 219–229.

Innerhofer, P.: Ein Regelmodell zur Analyse und Intervention in Familie und Schule. Z. klin. Psychol. 3 (1974), 1–29.

Iwert, H.: Ein Beitrag zur stationären psychologisch-heilpädagogischen Behandlung stotternder Kinder. Heilpäd. Forsch. 1(1964/1968) 231–243.

Jacobson, E.: Progressive Relaxation. University of Chicago Press, Chicago 1938.

Jasper, H.H.: A laboratory study of diagnostic indices of bilateral neuromuscular organization in stutterers and normal speakers. Psychol. Monogr. 48 (1932), 172–174.

Johnson, W. (Ed.): Stuttering in children and adults. Thirty years of research at the Univ. of Iowa. 2nd Ed. Univ. of Minnesota Press, Minneapolis 1956 (a).

Johnson, W.: The time, the place, and the problem. In. Johnson, W. (Ed.): Stuttering in children and adults. 2nd Ed. Univ. of Minnesota Press, Minneapolis 1956 (b), pp. 3–24.

Johnson, W.: A study of the onset and development of stuttering. In: Johnson, W. (Ed.): Stuttering in children and adults. 2nd Ed. Univ. of Minnesota Press, Minneapolis 1956 (c), pp. 37–73.

Johnson, W.: The onset of stuttering. University of Minnesota Press, Minneapolis 1959.

Johnson, W.: Measurement of oral reading and speaking rate and disfluency of adult male and female stutterers and nonstutterers. J. Speech Hear. Dis. 7 (1961), 1–20.

Johnson, W.: Stuttering. In: Johnson, W., Moeller, D. (Eds.): Speech handicapped school children. 3rd Ed. Harper & Row, New York 1967, pp. 229–329.

Johnson, W., Darley, F.L., Spriestersbach, D. C.: Diagnostic methods in speech pathology. Harper & Row, New York 1963.

Johnson, W., Knott, J.R.: Certain objective cues related to the precipitation of the moment of stuttering. J. Speech Dis. 2 (1937). 17–19.

Johnson, W., Moeller, D. (Eds.): Speech handicapped school children. 3rd Ed. Harper & Row, New York 1967.

Johnson, W., Rosen, L.: Effects of certain changes in speech patterns upon the frequency of stuttering. J. Speech Dis. 2 (1937) 101–104.

Jones, H.G.: Behavior therapy and stuttering: The need for a multivarious approach to a multiplex problem. In: Gray, B.B., England, G. (Eds.): Stuttering and the conditioning therapies. Monterey Institute for Speech and Hearing, Monterey 1969, pp. 187–197.

Jones, R.J., Arzrin, N.H.: Behavioral engineering: Stuttering as a function of stimulus duration during speech synchronization. J. Appl. Behav. Anal. 2 (1969), 223–229.

Jones, R.K.: Observations on stammering after localized cerebral injury. J. Neurol. Neurosurg. 29 (1966), 192–195.

Jones, R.K.: Dypraxic Ambiphasia—A neurophysiologic theory of stammering. Transact. Amer. neurol. Assoc. 92 (1967), 197–201.

Jussen, H.: Das Problem des Stotterns in der amerikanischen Fachliteratur. Die Sprachheilarbeit 2 (1964), 162–178.

Kanfer, F.H.: Selbstmanagement-Methoden. In: Kanfer, F.H., Goldstein, A.P. (Hrsg): Möglichkeiten der Verhaltensänderung. Urban & Schwarzenberg, München 1977, S. 350–406.

Karoly, P.: Operante Methoden. In: Kanfer, F.H., Goldstein, A.P. (Hrsg.): Möglichkeiten der Verhaltesänderung. Urban & Schwarzenberg, München 1977, S. 220–260.

Kehrer, H.E., Stegat, H.: Über die Behandlung von Stotterern nach verhaltenstherapeutischer Methode (negative Praxis). Prax. Kinderpsychol. Kinderpsychiat. 17 (1968), 164–170.

Keidel, W.D. (Hrsg.): Kurzefaßtes Lehrbuch der Physiologie. 4. Aufl. Thieme, Stuttgart 1975.

Kendrick, D.C.: The theory of »conditoned inhibition« as an exploration of negative practice effects: An experimental analysis. In: Eysenck, H.J. (Ed.): Behaviour therapy and the neuroses. Pergamon, Oxford 1960, pp. 221–235.

Kent, C.R.: The use of tranquilizers in the treatment of stuttering. J. Speech Dis. 28 (1963), 288.

Krech, H.: Das Entspannungstraining (ET). In: Jakobi, H. (Hrsg.): Phoniatrie. Barth, Leipzig 1963, S. 148–153.

Krugman, M.: Psychosomatic study of fifty stuttering children. J. Orthopsychiat. 16 (1946), 127–133.

Kuhlen, V.: Verhaltenstherapie im Kindesalter. Juventa, München 1972.

Kussmaul, A.: Die Störungen der Sprache. 4. Aufl. Vogel, Liepzig 1910.

Landolt, H., Luchsinger, R.: Sprachstörungen, Stottern und chronisch-organisches Psychosyndrom; elektroencephalographische Resultate und Untersuchungen der Sprache. Dtsch. med. Wschr. 79 (1954). 1012–1015.

Lebrun, Y., Bayle, M.: Surgery in the treatment of stuttering. In: Lebrun, Y., Hoops, R. (Eds.): Neurolinguistic approaches to stuttering. The Hague, Paris 1973, pp. 82–89.

Lebrun, Y., Hoops, R. (Eds.): Neurolinguistic approaches to stuttering. The Hague, Paris 1973.

Lee, B.S.: Artificial Stutter. J. Speech Hear. Dis. 16 (1951), 53–55.

Lefrancois, G.R.: Psychologie des Lernens. Springer, Berlin 1976.

Lehner, G.F.: Negative practice as a psychotherapeutic technique. In: Eysenck, H.J. (Eds.): Behaviour therapy and the neuroses. Pergamon, Oxford 1960, pp. 194–206.

Lenz, W.: Medizinische Genetik. 2. Aufl. Thieme, Stuttgart 1970.

Lieberman, M.A.: Gruppenmethoden. In: Kanfer, F.H., Goldstein, A.P. (Hrsg.): Möglichkeiten der Verhaltensänderung, Urban & Schwarzenberg. München 1977, S. 503–567.

Liebmann, A.: Stotternde Kinder. Steinnitz, Berlin 1903.

Liebmann, A.: Vorlesungen über Sprachstörungen. 9. Heft: Die psychische Behandlung von Sprachstörungen. Coblentz/Berlin 1914.

Linden, M., Manns, M.: Psychopharmakologie für Psychologen. Müller, Salzburg 1977.

Lombard: Contribution á la séméiologie de la surdité; un nouveau signe pour en dévoiler la simulation. Bull. Acad. Méd. 64 (1910), 127–130.

Lotzmann, G.: Zur Anwendung variierter Verzögerungszeiten bei Balbuties. Folia phoniat. 13 (1961), 276–312.

Luchsinger, R.: Über die Beziehungen der Sprache und Sprachstörungen zur sogenannten Feinmotorik. Folia phoniat. 1 (1948), 206–224.

Luchsinger, R.: Die Vererbung von Sprachund Stimmstörungen. Folia phoniat. 11 (1959), 7–64.

Lüking, P.: Die Symptome des Stotterns und ihre Registrierung. Die Sprachheilarbeit 2 (1957), 1–12.

Lüking, P.: Lautstreifen mit Prüfwerttafel und Merkblatt. 2. Aufl. Hrsg.: Arbeitsgem. Sprachheilpäd. Dtschl. Hamburg 1960.

Macioszek, G.: Die verzögerte akustische Rückmeldung bei Stotterern mit unterschiedlichem Ausmaß der Störung, Z. klin. Psychol. 2 (1973), 278–299.

MacKay, D.G.: Metamorphosis of a critical interval: Age-linked changes in the delay in auditory feedback that produces maximal disruption of speech. J. Acoust. Soc. Amer. 19 (1968), 811–821.

MacLaren, J.: The treatment of stammering by the Cherry-Sayers method: Clinical impressions. In: Eysenck, H.J. (Ed.): Behaviour therapy and the neuroses. Pergamon, Oxford 1960, pp. 457–460.

Mahaffey, R.B., Stromsta, C.: Effects of peak-clipped and center-clipped delayed sidetone. J. Amer. Speech Hear. Ass. 7 (1965), 413–414.

Mahoney, M.J., Thoresen, C.E. (Eds.): Self-control: Power to the person. Brooks/Cole, Monterey 1974.

Manns, M.: Verhaltenstherapie des Stotterns. In: Duhm, E. (Hrsg.): Praxis der Klinischen Pschologie, Band I. Hogrefe, Göttingen 1969, S. 180–199.

Maraist, J.A., Hutton, C.: Effects of auditory masking upon the speech of stutterers. J. Speech Hear. Dis. 22 (1957), 385–389.

Marks, M.: Stuttering viewed as a sequence of responses. In: Gray, B.B., England, G. (Eds.): Stuttering and the conditioning therapies. Monterey Institute for Speech and Hearing, Monterey 1969, pp. 29–39.

Martin, R.R.: The experimental manipulation of stuttering behaviors. In: Sloane, H.N., McAulay, B.D. (Eds.): Operant procedures in remedial speech and language training. Houghton-Mifflin, Boston 1968, pp. 325–347.

Martin, R.R., Siegel, G.M.: The effects of response contingent shock on stuttering. J. Speech Hear. Res. 9 (1966), 340–352.

Martyn, M.M., Sheehan, J.G.: Onset of stuttering and recovery. Behav. Res. Ther. 6 (1968), 295–307.

May, A.E., Hackwood, A.: Some effects of masking and eliminating low frequency feedback on the speech of stutterers. Behav. Res. Ther. 6 (1966), 219–224.

McCroskey, R.L.: The relative contribution of auditory and tactile cues to certain aspects of speech. South. Speech J. 24 (1958), 84–90.

McDearmont, J.R.: Primary stuttering at the onset of stuttering: A re-examination of the data. J. Speech Hear. Res. 11 (1968), 631–637.

McIntyre, M.E., Silverman, F.H., Trotter, W.D.: Transcendental meditation and stuttering: A preliminary report. Percept. Mot. Skills 39 (1974), 294.

Meichenbaum, D.: Methoden der Selbstinstruktion. In: Kanfer, F.H., Goldstein, A.P. (Hrsg.): Möglichkeiten der Verhaltensänderung. Urban & Schwarzenberg. München 1977, S. 407–450.

Meyer, V., Mair, J.M.: A new technique to control stammering: A preliminary report. Behav. Res. Ther. 1 (1963) 251–254.

Milisen, R.L., Johnson, W.: A comparative study of stutterers. Archives of Speech 1 (1936) 61–86.

Miller, N.E.: Comments on theoretical models illustrated by the development of a theory of conflict behavior. J. Pers. 20 (1951), 81–100.

Moore, W.H., Ritterman, S.I.: The effects of response contingent reinforcement and response contingent punishment upon the frequency of stuttered verbal behavior. Behav. Res. Ther. 11 (1973), 43–48.

Morley, M.E.: Development and disorders of speech in childhood. Livingstone, Edinburgh 1957.

Morris, R.J.: Methoden der Angstreduktion. In: Kanfer, F.H., Goldstein A.P. (Hrsg): Möglichkeiten der Verhaltensänderung. Urban & Schwarzenberg, München 1977, S. 261–308.

Motsch, M., Affeld-Niemeyer, P., Bader, L., Hoefert, H.: Zur Analyse der Interaktion von stotternden Kindern und ihren Eltern. In: Verhaltenstherapie—Praxis. Kongreßberichte 1976. Sonderheft II/77 der Deutschen Gesellschaft für Verhaltenstherapie, Postfach 1343, 7400 Tübingen 1977.

Mowrer, O.H., Two-factor learning theory reconsidered, with special reference to secondary reinforcement and the concept of habit. Psychol. Rev. 63 (1956), 114–128.

Mowrer, O.H.: A résumé of basic principles of learning. In: Gregory, H.H. (Ed.): Learning theory and stuttering therapy. Northwestern Univ. Press, Evanston 1968, pp. 3–20.

Mückenhoff, E.: Rhythmisch-signalgebundenes Sprechen als methodisches Hilfsmittel in der Sotterertherapie. Z. Heilpäd. 1976 (Heft 1), S. 39–42.

Murphy, A.T., Fitzsimons, R.M.: Stuttering and personality dynamics. Ronald, New York 1960.

Mysak, E.D.: Servo-theory and stuttering. J. Speech Hear. Dis. 15 (1960), 188–195.

Nadoleczny, M.: Kurzes Lehrbuch der Sprach- und Stimmheilkunde mit besonderer Berücksichtigung des Kindesalters. Vogel, Leipzig 1926.

Neeley, J.A.: A study of speech behavior of stutterers and nonstutterers under normal and delayed auditory feedback. J. Speech Hear. Dis. 7 (1961), 63–83.

Nelson, S.E., Hunter, N., Walter, M.: Stuttering in twin types. J. Speech Dis. 10 (1945), 335–343.

Nessel, E.: Die verzögerte Sprachrückkoppelung (Lee-Effekt) bei Stotternden. Folia phoniat. 10 (1958), 199–204.

Ockel, H.H.: Zum Problem des Stotterns. Prax. Kinderpsychol. Kinderpsychiat. 6 (1959), 213–223.

Orthmann, W., Scholz, H.J.: Stottern. Kompendium. Marhold, Berlin 1975.

Oxtoby, E.T.: Frequency of stuttering in relation to induced modifications following expectancy of stuttering. In: Johnson, W. (Ed.): Stuttering in children and adults, 2nd Ed. University of Minnesota Press, Minneapolis 1956, pp. 218–225.

Parker, C.S., Christopherson, F.: Electronic aid in the treatment of stammer. Med. Electr. Biol. Eng. 1 (1963), 121–125.

Peachers, W.C., Harris, W.E.: Speech disorders in World War II: Stuttering. J. Speech Dis. 11 (1946), 303–308.

Perkins, W.H.: Stuttering: Some common denominators. In: Barbara, D.A. (Ed.): New directions in stuttering. Thomas, Springfield 1965.

Perkins, W.H.: Replacement of stuttering with normal speech: I. Rationale. J. Speech Hear. Dis. 38 (1973a), 283–294.

Perkins, W.H.: Replacement of stuttering with normal speech: II. Clinical procedures. J. Speech Hear. Dis. 38 (1973b), 295–303.

Perkins, W.H., Curlee, R.F.: Clinical impressions of portable masking unit effects in stuttering. J. Speech Hear. Dis. 34 (1969), 360–362.

Perkins, W.H., Haugen, C.: The relationship between frequency of stuttering and open expression of aggression. Paper, read before meeting of Amer. Speech Hear. Assoc. 1965. Zitiert nach Van Riper (1971).

Perkins, W.H., Rudas, J., Johnson, L., Michael, W.B., Curlee, R.F.: Replacement of stuttering with normal speech: III. Clinical effectiveness. J. Speech Hear. Dis. 39 (1974), 414–428.

Quarrington, B.: Cyclic variations in stuttering frequency and severity and some related forms of variations. Canad, J. Psychol. 10 (1956), 179–184.

Quarrington, B.: Stuttering as a function of the information value and sentence position of words. J. abnorm. soc. Psychol. 70 (1965), 221–224.

Rawnsley, A.F., Harris, J.D.: Comparative analysis of normal speech and speech with delayed sidetone by means of sound spectograms. USN Submar. Med. Res. Lab. Rep. 13 (1954), No. 248.

200   STUTTERING: INTEGRATING THEORY AND PRACTICE

Richter, E.: Rhythmus als ausdrucksfördernder Faktor in der Übungsbehandlung des Stotterns. Die Sprachheilarbeit 12 (1967), 50–60.

Richter, E.: Über die Fremd- und Selbststeuerung in der Therapie des Stotterns. Die Sprachheilarbeit 15 (1970), 161–170.

Richter, E.: Kritische Überlegungen zu den mangelnden Heilerfolgen in der Behandlung des Stotterns. Z. Heilpäd. 12 (1972), 863–876.

Rickard, H.C., Mundy, M.B.: Direct manipulation of stuttering behavior: An experimental-clinical approach. In: Ullman, L.P., Krasner, L. (Hrsg.): Case studies in behavior modification. Holt, Rinehart & Winston, New York 1965, pp. 268–274.

Rieber, R.W.: Stuttering and self-concept. J. Psychol. 55 (1963), 307–311.

Rieber, R.W.: Word magic, self-alienation and stuttering. Folia phoniat. 17 (1965), 202–216.

Ringel, R.L., Steer, M.D.: Some effects of tactile and auditory alteration on speech output. J. Speech. Hear. Res. 6 (1963), 369–378.

Röck, E.: Verzögerte auditive Rückkoppelung (VAR) der Lautsprache. In: Röck, E. (Hrsg.): Verzögerte Auditive Rückkoppelung (VAR). Huber, Bern 1977, S. 13–74.

Rosenthal, T.L.: Severe stuttering and maladjustment treated by desensitization and social influence. Behav. Res. Ther. 6 (1968), 125–130.

Rosenzweig, M.R.: Representations of the two ears at the auditory cortex. Amer. J. Physiol. 167 (1951), 147–158.

Russel, J.C., Clark. A.W., Van Sommers. P.: Treatment of stammering by reinforcement of fluent speech. Behav. Res. Ther. 6 (1968), 447–453.

Sandler, J.: Aversive Methoden. In: Kanfer, F.H., Goldstein, A.P. (Hrsg.): Möglichkeiten der Verhaltensänderung. Urban & Schwarzenberg. München 1977, S. 309–349.

Santostefano, S.: Anxiety and hostility in stuttering. J. Speech Hear. Res. 3 (1960), 337–347.

Schilling, A.: Die Behandlung des Stotterns. Folia phoniat. 17 (1965), 365–458.

Schilling, A., Krüger, W.: Untersuchungen über die Motorik sprachgestörter Kinder. HNO 8 (1959/60), 205–209.

Schliesser, H.F., Coleman, R.O.: Effectiveness of certain procedures for alterations of auditory and oral tactile sensation of speech. Percept. Mot. Skills 26 (1968), 275–281.

Schmidt, B., Standop, R.: Die Bedeutung von Selbstkonfrontation, Sozialtraining und Therapiehäufigkeit bei der Verhaltensmodifikation erwachsener Stotternder. Unveröff. Diplomarbeit, Münster 1974.

Schmidt, H.: Ein Beitrag zur Differentialdiagnose Stottern: Poltern. Die Sprachheilarbeit 14 (1969), 105–112.

Schmoigl, S., Ladisich, W.: EEG-Untersuchungen bei Stotterern. Folia phoniat. 19 (1967), 359–367.

Schneider, E.: Über das Stottern. Ursache, Entstehung, Verlauf und Heilung. Beiheft Nr. 22; Schweiz. Z. Psychol. Anw. 1953.

Schönhärl, E., Bente, D.: Veränderungen im EEG bei Stottern. Kongreßbericht, Gemeinschaftstagung allg. angew. Phonetik; Hamburg-Altona 1960, 82–87.

Schulte, D.: Ein Schema für Diagnose und Therapieplanung in der Verhaltenstherapie. In: Schulte, D. (Hrsg.): Diagnostik in der Verhaltenstherapie. Urban & Schwarzenberg, München 1974, S. 75–104.

Schulte, D., Kemmler, L.: Systematische Beobachtung in der Verhaltenstherapie. In: Schulte, D. (Hrsg.): Diagnostik in der Verhaltenstherapie. Urban & Schwarzenberg, München 1974, S. 152–195.

Schultheis, J.R.: Tiefenpsychologische Aspekte des Stotterns. Die Sprachheilarbeit 16 (1971), 70–83.

Schultz, I.H.: Übungsheft für das autogene Training. 14. Aufl. Thieme, Stuttgart 1969.

Schulze, C.: Methoden der Stotterbehandlung bei Kindern. In: Brengelmann, J.C., Tunner, W. (Hrsg.): Behaviour Therapy—Verhaltenstherapie. Urban & Schwarzenberg, München 1973, S. 135–142.

Schulze, C.: Kann Biofeedback Stottervorläufer kontrollieren? Sonderheft I/1978 der Deutschen Gesellschaft für Verhaltenstherapie, Postfach 1343, 74 Tübingen (1978), 234–245.

Schwartz, M.F.: Stottern ist heilbar. Econ, Düsseldorf 1977.

Seeman, M.: Über somatische Befunde beim Stottern. Mschr. Ohrenheilk. 68 (1934) 895–912.

Seeman, M.: Sprachstörungen bei Kindern. Volk und Gesundheit, Berlin 1969.

Shames, G.H.: Dysfluency and stuttering. Pediat. Clin. N. Amer. 15 (1968), 691–704.

Shames, G.H., Egolf, D.B.: Operant conditioning and the management of stuttering. Prentice-Hall, Englewood Cliffs 1976.

Shames, G.H., Sherrick, C.E.: A discussion of nonfluency and stuttering as operant behavior. J. Speech Hear. Dis. 28 (1963), 3–18.

Shearer. W.M.: A theoretical consideration of the self-concept and body image in stuttering therapy. J. Amer. Speech Hear. Assoc. 3 (1961), 115 (abstract).

Shearer, W.M., Simmons, F.B.: Middle ear activity during speech in normal speakers and stutterers. J. Speech Hear. Res. 8 (1965), 203–207.

Sheehan, J.G.: The modification of stuttering through non-reinforcement. J. abnorm. soc. Psychol. 46 (1951), 51–63.

Sheehan, J.G.G.: Theory and treatment of stuttering as an approach-avoidance conflict. J. Psychol. 36 (1953), 27–49.

Sheehan, J.G.: Self-perception in stuttering. J. clin. Psychol. 10 (1954), 70–72.

Sheehan, J.G.: Conflict theory of stuttering. In: Eisenson, J. (Ed.): Stuttering: A symposium. Harper, New York 1958, pp. 121–166.

Sheehan, J.G.: Cyclic variation in stuttering: Comment of Taylor and Taylors »Test of predictions from the conflict hypothesis of stuttering«. J. abnorm. Psychol. 74 (1969), 452–453.

Sheehan, J.G. (Ed.): Stuttering. Research and therapy. Harper & Row, New York 1970 (a).

Sheehan, J.G.: Research frontiers in stuttering. In: Sheehan, J. G. (Ed.): Stuttering. Research and therapy. Harper & Row, New York 1970 (b), pp. 312–350.

Sheehan, J.G.: Role-conflict theory. In: Sheehan, J.G. (Ed.): Stuttering. Research and Therapy. Harper & Row, New York 1970 (c), pp. 2–35.

Sheehan, J.G.: Role therapy. In: Sheehan, J.G. (Ed.): Stuttering. Research and therapy. Harper & Row, New York 1970 (d), pp. 260–311.

Sheehan, J.G., Martyn, M.M.: Spontaneous recovery from stuttering. J. Speech Hear. Res. 9 (1966), 121–135.

Sheehan, J.G., Martyn, M.M.: Methodology in studies of recovery from stuttering. J. Speech Hear. Res. 10 (1967), 396–400.

Shulman, E.: Factors influencing the variability of stuttering. In: Johnson, W. (Ed.): Stuttering in children and adults. 2nd Ed. Univ. of Minnesota Press, Minneapolis 1956, pp. 207–217.

Siegel, G.M.: Punishment, stuttering and disfluency. J. Speech Hear. Res. 13 (1970), 677–714.

Siegel, G.M., Martin, R.R.: Verbal punishment of disfluencies during spontaneous speech. Language and Speech 10 (1967), 244–251.

Siegel, G.M., Martin, R.R.: The effects of verbal stimuli on disfluencies during spontaneous speech. J. Speech Hear. Res. 11 (1968), 358–364.

Sieland, B., Schäuble, W.: Training und Transfer. In: Sader, M., Schäuble, W., Theis, W. (Hrsg.): Verbesserung von Interaktion durch Gruppendynamik. Aschendorff, Münster 1976, S. 129–170.

Smith, K.U.: Delayed sensory feedback and behavior. Saunders, Philadelphia 1962.

Smith, K.U., Smith, W.M.: Perception and motion. Saunders, Philadelphia 1962.

Smith, K.U., Tierney, D.: Delayed speech feedback and age. J. Speech Hear. Res. 14 (1971), 214–219.

Soderberg, G.A.: Delayed auditory feedback and stuttering. J. Speech Hear. Dis. 33 (1968), 260–267.

Soderberg, G.A.: Delayed auditory feedback and the speech of stutterers. A review of studies. J. Speech Hear. Dis. 34 (1969), 20–29.

Stange, G.: Erziehung, Bildung und Therapie stotternder Kinder in einem Kinderheim. Beiheft 1; Die Sonderschule 1970.

Stassi, E.J.: Disfluency of normal speakers and reinforcement. J. Speech Hear. Res. 5 (1962), 272–283.

Stier, E.: Untersuchungen über Linkshändigkeit und die funktionellen Differenzen der Hirnhälften. Fischer, Jena 1911.

Stromsta, C.: The effects of altering the fundamental frequency of masking on the speech performance of stutterers. Techn. Rep., Nat. Inst. Health 1958.

Stromsta, C.: Experimental blockage of phonation by distorted sidetone. J. Speech Hear. Res. 2 (1959), 286–301.

Stromsta, C.: Interaural phase disparity of stutterers and nonstutterers. J. Speech Hear. Res. 15 (1972), 771–780.

Sutton, S., Chase, R.A.: White noise and stuttering. J. Speech Hear. Res. 4 (1961), 72.

Tate, M.W., Cullinan, W.L.: Measurement of consistency of stuttering. J. Speech Hear. Res. 5 (1962), 272–283.

Taylor, I.: What words are stuttered. Psychol. Bull. 65 (1966), 233–245.

Thoresen, C.E., Mahoney, M.J.: Behavioral self-control. Holt, Rinehart & Winston, New York 1974.

Tiffany, W.R., Hanley, C.: Adaptation to delayed sidetone. J. Speech Hear. Dis. 21 (1956), 164–172.

Tomatis, A.: Recherches sur la Pathologie du Bégaiement. Journ. Franc. ORL 3 (1954), 384–390.

Tomatis, A.: L'Oreille et le Langage. Éditions du Seuil, Paris 1963.

Travis, L.E.: Speech Pathology. Appleton-Century, New York 1931.

Travis, L.E. (Ed.): Handbook of speech pathology. Appleton, New York 1957.

Trotter, W.D., Lesch, M.M.: Personal experiences with a stutter-aid. J. Speech Hear. Dis. 32 (1967), 270–272.

Trotter, W.D., Silverman, F.A.: Does the effect of pacing speech with a miniature metronome on stuttering wear off? Percept. Mot. Skills 39 (1974), 429–430.

Tunner, W.: Verhaltensmodifikationen bei Sprechstörungen. In: Brengelmann J.C., Tunner, W. (Hrsg.): Behaviour Therapy—Verhaltenstherapie. Urban & Schwarzenberg, München 1973, S. 128–134.

Tunner, W.: Analyse und Modifikation des Stotterns. In: Kraiker, Ch. (Hrsg.): Handbuch der Verhaltenstherapie. Kindler, München 1974, S. 445–464.

Tunner, W.: Angst bei neurotischen Sprechstörungen: Diagnose und Therapie. In: Störungen der Sprachentwicklung. Tagungsbericht Nürnberg 1976 der Dtsch. Ges. Sprachheilpäd. Wartenberg, Hamburg 1976, S. 153–160.

Tunner, W., Bruckmoser: Reizkontrolle bei der Behandlung des Stotterns. Mitteilungen der Gesellschaft zur Förderung der Verhaltenstherapie, Heft 2/3, 1969, S. 6–7.

Tunner, W., Florin, I: Lernpsychologische Überlegungen zur Genese und Therapie des Stotterns. Mitteilungen der Gesellschaft zur Förderung der Verhaltenstherapie, Heft 2/3, 1969, S. 20–26.

Ullrich de Muynck, R., Ullrich R.: Einübung von Selbstvertrauen und sozialer Kompetenz. I bis III. Pfeiffer, München 1977.

Van Dantzig, M.: Syllable-Tapping: A new method for the help of stammerers. J. Speech Dis. 5 (1940), 127–132.

Van Dusen, D.: A laterality study of non-stutterers and stutterers. J. Speech Dis. 4 (1939), 261–265.

Van Riper, C.: Experiments in stuttering therapy. In: Eisenson, J. (Ed.): Stuttering. A symposium. Harper, New York 1958.

Van Riper, C.: Speech correction: Principles and methods. Prentice-Hall, Engelwood-Cliffs 1963.

Van Riper, C.: Stuttering and cluttering. The differential diagnosis. Folia phoniat. 22 (1970), 347–353.

Van Riper, C.: The nature of stuttering. Prentice-Hall, Englewood-Cliffs 1971.

Van Riper, C: The treatment of stuttering. Prentice-Hall, Englewood-Cliffs 1973.

Van Riper, C., Hull, C.J.: The quantitative measurement of the effect of certain situations on stuttering. In: Johnson, W. (Ed.): Stuttering in children and adults. 2nd Ed. Univ. of Minnesota Press, Minneapolis 1956, pp. 199–206.

Vlassova, N.A.: Die Therapie des Stotterns bei Kindern. Kongreßbericht. Intern. Arbeitst. über Fragen der Rehab., Dispensoirebetreuung und Prämorbidität. Thieme, Leipzig 1958, S. 699–701.

Wada, J., Rasmussen, T.: Intracarotic injection of Sodium Amytol for the lateralization of cerebral speech dominance. J. Neurosurg. 7 (1960), 266–282.

Wallen, V.: Primary stuttering in a twenty-eight-year-old adult. J. Speech Hear. Dis. 26 (1961), 394.

Wallrabenstein, F.: Sprachheilpädagogik (Logopädie) als Aufgabe der Gesundheitserziehung. Hrsg. Bundesverband für gesundheitliche Volkserziehung, Bad Godesberg 1963.

Walton, D., Black, D.A.: The application of learning theory to the treatment of stammering. In: Eysenck, H.J. (Ed.): Behaviour therapy and the neuroses. Pergamon, Oxford 1960, pp. 123–134.

Walton, D., Mather, M.D.: The relevance of generalization techniques to the treatment of stammering and phobic symptoms. Behav. Res. Ther. 1 (1963), 121–125.

204 STUTTERING: INTEGRATING THEORY AND PRACTICE

Watzlawik, P.: Die Möglichkeit des Andersseins. Huber, Bern 1977.

Webster, R.L., Dorman, M.F.: Decreases in stuttering frequency as a function of continuous and contingent forms of auditory masking. J. Speech Hear. Res. 13 (1970), 82–86.

Webster, R.L., Lubker. B.B.: Masking of auditory feedback in stutterers speech. J. Speech Hear. Res. 11 (1968), 221–223.

Weiss, D.A.: Der Zusammenhang zwischen Poltern und Stottern. Folia phoniat. 4 (1950), 252–262.

Weiss, D.A.: Cluttering. Prentice-Hall, Englewood-Cliffs 1964.

Weiss, D.A.: Similarities and differences between cluttering and stuttering. Folia phoniat. 19 (1967), 98–104.

Wendlandt, W.: Resozialisierung erwachsener Stotternder. Marhold, Berlin 1972.

Wendlandt, W.: Selbstbehauptungstraining—ein verhaltenstherapeutischer Ansatz in der Behandlung erwachsener Stotternder. Z. klin. Psychol. Psychoth. 22 (1974), 236–246.

Wendlandt, W.: Rollenspiele zur Verhaltensmodifikation—Ansätze für dies pädagogische Praxis. In: Verhaltenstherapie—Praxis, Kongreßberichte 1976, Sonderheft II/77 der Deutschen Gesellschaft für Verhaltenstherapie, Postfach 1343, 74 Tübingen 1977, S. 41–58.

Wendlandt, W., Hoefert, H.W.: Selbstsicherheitstraining. Müller, Salzburg 1976.

Wengle, M.E.: Die systematische Desensibilisierung. In: Kraiker, Ch. (Hrsg.): Handbuch der Verhaltenstherapie. Kindler, München 1974, S. 279–324.

Wepman, J.M.: Familial incidence in stammering. J. Speech Dis. 4 (1939), 199–204.

Wertheimer, M.: Drei Abhandlungen zur Gestalttheorie. Erlangen 1925.

West, R.: An agnostic's speculation about stuttering. In: Eisenson, J. (Ed.): Stuttering. A symposium. Harper & Row, New York 1958, S. 167–221.

Westrich, E.: Der Stotterer. Psychologie und Therapie. Dürrsche Buchhandlung, Bonn-Bad Godesberg 1971.

Westrich, E.: Sprach- und Sprechstörungen (Sprachbehinderungen). In: Handbuch der Psychologie, 8. Band, Klinische Psychologie. 2. Halbband (Hrsg. L. Pongratz). Hogrefe, Göttingen 1978, S. 2372–2420.

Widlak, H.: Modifikation des Stotterns durch negative Praxis. Phil. Diss. Münster 1977.

Widlak, H., Fiedler, P.A.: Einige Überlegungen zur Früherkennung und Frühbehandlung kindlichen Stotterns. In: Verhaltenstherapie—Praxis. Kongreßberichte 1976. Sonderheft II/77 der Deutschen Gesellschaft für Verhaltenstherapie, Postfach 1343, 74 Tübingen 1977, S. 210–222.

Williams, D.E.: A point of view about stuttering. J. Speech Hear. Dis. 22 (1957), 390–397.

Winkelmann, N.W.: Chlorpromazine in the treatment of neuropsychiatric disorders. J. Amer. med. Ass. 155 (1954), 18–21.

Wischner, G.J.: Experimental approach to expectancy and anxiety in stuttering behavior. J. Speech Hear. Dis. 17 (1952), 139–154.

Wolpe, J.: Psychotherapy by reciprocal inhibition. Stanford Univ. Press, Stanford 1958.

Wyneken, C.: Über das Stottern und dessen Heilung. Z. rat. Med. 31 (1868), 1–29.

Yates, A.J.: Delayed auditory feedback. Psychol. Bull. 60 (1963a), 213–232.

Yates, A.J.: Recent empirical and theoretical approaches to experimental and manipulation of speech in normal subjects and in stammerers. Behav. Res. Ther. 1 (1963b), 95–119.

Yates, A.J.: Behavior Therapy. Wiley, New York 1970.

Zimmer, D.: Ausbildung sozialer Kompetenz durch Training in Verhaltensgeschicklichkeit und Selbstregulation. Phil. Diss. Münster 1976.

Zopf, R., Motsch, M.: Eine logopädisch-psychologische Gruppentherapie erwachsener Stotternder. Die Sprachheilarbeit 18 (1973), 143–148.

Zuckrigl, H. und A., Helbling, H.: Rhythmik hilft Behinderten. Ziele und Realisationsbeispiele der rhythmischen Erziehung behinderter Kinder. Reinhardt, München 1976.

Index

A

Activity, to reduce symptoms, 65
Adaptation effect, 7, 9-10, 63
  age and, 10
  in diagnosis, 78
  environment and, 9
  spontaneous recovery and, 10
Age
  adaptation and, 10
  of onset, 16
  therapy and, 162, 181
Alcohol, effect on stuttering, 12
Ambidexterity, in stutterers, 24
Anticipatory effect, 8
Anticipatory aversive stimuli, 106
Anxiety
  conditioned tension and, 34
  conflict and, 49
  management, 133
  overcoming, 52, 167
  with parents, 50
  -producing stimuli, 41-42
  punishment and, 107
  from social sources, 134, 151
  tape recordings and, 128
Articulation drills, 101
Assessment
  See also Diagnosis

of experiences, 82
motor-physiological, 75-78
of speech disorder, 74-75
stimulus, 81
Associated movements, in
  development, 39
Attitude
  age and, 174
  changes during therapy, 180
  of stutterers, 140-141
Auditory control, of speech, 56,
  29-30, 60, 62, 79, 89, 104, 108
  cognitive basis for, 62
  therapy and, 139-140
Auditory debility, from hemisphere
  dominance, 25-26
Auditory feedback, 126
  interferences by, 126
  masking, 112
  speech control and, 58
Autogenic training, 133
Azrin, N.H. and Nunn, R.G., "rapid
  therapy program," 125

B

Balbutiogram, 74-75
Beech, H.R. and Fransella, F.,
  cluttering vs. stuttering, 7

Note: Italicized numbers include references to tables and figures.

Behavior
  affective, 51
  assessment, 82
  avoidance, 43, 61, 122
  cognitive control, 51, 91-92
  conspicuous, 119-120
  escape, 61
  improvement, 179
  learned, 38, 55, 149
    testing, 155-156
  methods of therapy and, 175
  operant, 38, 90-91
  regulation, 82-83
  reinforcers, 106
  respondent control, 90
  social, 43-46, 175
    disorders in, 149
    learned, 149
    in therapy groups, 156
  somatic and environmental
    factors, 37
  stability, after therapy, 182
  symptomatic, 86
  theories, 38-40
  of therapist, 177
  therapeutic interventions and, 67
Behavior therapy, 100, 128, 137, 150,
  170, 184
  combination of methods, 174
  resocialization, 175-176
  role playing and, 151-152
  as stuttering therapy, 106
Biofeedback
  to improve breathing, 131-132
  devices, 133
Bloodstein, O.
  activities to reduce symptoms, 11
  punishment, 107
  stuttering development, 17-18
"Blowing technique," 130-133
  self-responsibility and, 142
Bluemel, C.S., stuttering development,
  17
Böhme, G., theory of
  "multidimensional therapy," 169
Brain Damage, 84

Brain injuries, as cause, 22
Breathing, 4, 6, 33, 171, 174
  aids, 169
  behavior, 170
  exercises, 175
  inspirational speech, 6
  irregularities, 131-132
  modification, 104-105
  practice, 172
  relaxation and, 132
  residual air speech, 6
  self-responsibility and, 142
  speaking and, 40, 101
  in therapy, 153
Bruten, E.J. and Shoemaker, D.J.,
  theory of classical conditioning
  and stuttering, 40

C

Calavrezo, C., theory of speech
  gestures, 5, 103-104, 164
Caretakers
  See also Parents
  role in therapy, 157-158
Casual factors, 3, 84-85
Central nervous system, and speech
  musculature, 56
Cerebral disfunction, and
  psychomotor training, 165
Cerebral dominance, and speech
  disorders, 23-26
Cerebral motor disturbances, with
  stuttering, 22
Children, 12, 15, 17-20
  ego and, 50
  success of therapy in, 181
  teasing, 44
  therapist's attitude and, 127
Churchill, Winston, 6
Classical conditioning, 40
Clinical phenomena, 3
Clonic stuttering, 4, 15, 75
  remission in, 13
  as stammering, 4

-tonic stuttering, 4
Cluttering
   defined, 7
   stuttering vs., 6, 7, 11, 87, 88
Cognitive-affective experiences, 82
Cognitive aspects, 62, 81-83
Cognitive restructuring, 140, 141
Cognitive social aspects, 46-47, 66
Competence, expectancies, 82
Conditioning. *See* Behavior
Conflict
   avoidance, 51
   affecting behavior, 163
   as cause of stuttering, 46-47
   defense mechanisms and, 50
   emotional vs. physical, 49
   intrapersonal bases, 47-48, 92
   origins, 49-50
   parents and, 50
   social, and role playing, 152
   talking vs. not talking, 47
Consistency effect, 7-9, 63
   in diagnosis, 78
Constitutional aspects. *See*
   Neurophysiological aspects
Contingent aversive stimuli, 106
Continuity hypothesis, 38
Control. *See* Self-Control
Cure mythology, 186
Cybernetic approaches, 56

D

Deafness, 30
"Dehydration therapy," 99
Delayed auditory feedback (DAF),
   27, 64, 174
   devices, 113
   diverting conditions, 30
   masking conditions and, 30
   research using, 31-32
   sex differences and, 114
   speech-disturbing effects, 28
   symptom reduction by, 30
   in therapy, 112-114, 139, 142, 175

Depth psychology, 49-51, 99, 178
Desensitization
   (in sensu), 133-134
   (in vivo), 134
   systematic, 174-175
   in therapy, 175
Development, 18-20
   hypotheses, 39
   normal, 85
   stages, 17
Developmental stuttering, 56, 58,
   162-163
   spontaneous remissions, 16
Diagnosis
   See also Assessment
   as cause of stuttering, 65-66
   data collection, 74-75
   therapy and, 71-73
Diagnosogenic theory, 43
Dialogue, in therapy, 176-178
Differential diagnosis, 87
Distinctive cognitive organization, 46
Downton, W., breathing theory, 131
Drugs, in therapy, 134-135, 170

E

Electroencephalogram, of stutterers
   vs. nonstutterers, 22-23
Embolophones *(Embolophonien),* 5,
   77
   See also Patching
Embolophrases *(Embolophrasien),* 5,
   77
Environmental factors, 37, 100
   in auditory control, 60, 61
   control of, 148
Epilepsy, 23
Evaluation, of therapy results, 147
Exercises, in therapy, 143-144, 175
Eye contact, with stutterer, 5

F

Fear
   as cause of stuttering, 40, 43
   leading to helplessness, 45

overcoming, 145-146, 167, 170
of reactions of others, 177
of talking, 50, 170
of social rejection, 44
Fernau-Horn, H., age adapted
therapy, 171
Fiedler, P.A., classification for
assessment, 81-83
Flicklaute, 5
See also Patching
Flickwörter, 5
Froeschels, E., developmental stages,
15-16, 17
Functional behavior theory. *See*
Operant conditioning; Classical
conditioning

G

"General activation syndrome," 65, 92
German synonyms for "stuttering," 3
Gestures
speech, 78-79, 126, 131, 164, 165
in therapy, 153
Gesture language, 142-143
Gutzmann, A.,
"breathing" method, 104
"speaking the vowel," 101
Gutzmann, Jr., H., therapeutic
methods, 102
Gutzmann, Sr., H., therapeutic
methods, 101-102

H

Haptometronome, 115, 142, 172
Helplessness
feeling of, 45, 50, 65
overcoming, 167
recordings and, 128
Hereditary factors, 21-22, 61-62, 85
twins, 21-22, 61
Historical references, 99-100

I

Identification, early, 162-163
Identity, 51
Imitation, 60
"Inhibition therapy," 174-175
Inspirational speech, 6
Institutionalization, 97
Internal causes, 100
Internal sensory processes, 51
Iteration, 88-89

J

Johnson, W.
avoidance behavior, 43
diagnosis as cause, 65-66, 162
onset, 16
speech development in stutterers
vs. nonstutterers, 42
Jones' hypotheses, 25

K

Kinesthetic feedback, 58, 61
Knowledge gaps, 149

L

Labeling, 3, 12, 18
Laryngospasm, 40
blowing technique and, 104
as cause of stuttering, 33
Learning theory, 38
Lee Effect, The, 27-28
"negative," 30
and delayed auditory feedback,
114
Liebmann, A., "unisono method,"
170
Logopedic approaches, 99, 175
Lüking, P., balbutiogram, 74

M

Maintenance of stuttering hypotheses,
39
Management of stuttering, 3
See also Therapy
comprehensive, 101
Masking, 112, 142
devices, 112
Metronomes, 142, 172
use with children, 165
to control speech, 114-118, 130
in paced speech, 132
Micronome, 115, 142
Miller, N. E., conflict model, *47-48*
Mimicking, 5, 78, 126, 131
video recordings and, 130
Morphemes, in therapy, 102
Motor aphasia, 24
Motor activities, in overcoming
speech block, 11
"Motor clumsiness," 164
Motor-physiological characteristics,
75-76
Mowrer, O.H., 2 Factor Theory, 42
Muscles
involved in stuttering, 4
relaxation of, 101, 133
tension, 33
Music therapy, 99

N

Narcotics, 12
Negative practice, 108-110, 142,
174-175
"Nervous habit," 120
Nervousness, as cause of stuttering,
44
Neuromuscular discoordination
psychological factors, 34
as stuttering, 33-34
Neurophysiological aspects, 59
Neuropsychological aspects, 48-49,
89, 100, 104, 108, 138-139

Neuropsychological model, *56-58*
Neuropsychological propositions, 139
"Normal" stuttering, 56

O

Onset, 84
gradual vs. sudden, 16-17
Operant conditioning, 105-106
Operant learning process, 42, 107-108
Oral motor patterns, 76
Organic variables, 22-30, 83-84, 86
Origin hypotheses, 38

P

Paced speech, 126
"Paradoxical breathing" (*Paradoxen
Atemtyp*), 6, 131
Parakinesis, 5, 103, 132
Parakinetics, in diagnosis, 78
Parents, 59, 60
See also Caretakers
–child interaction, 163
as cotherapists, 97, 163-164, 168
early identification by, 162-163
reactions, 66, 127
rearing practices, 49-50
social pressure on, 65
as therapists, 165-166
as therapeutic aides, 107
Patching, 5
Patterns, of stuttering, 7-10
Pedagogical approaches, 99
Perception, disturbed, 26
Perceptive awareness, as cause of
stuttering, 110
Perceptual defect, as cause of
stuttering, 32-33
Phi test, 25
Phonemes, in therapy, 102
Physiological concomitants,
assessment of, 76

Physiological stuttering, 7
  See also Developmental stuttering
  symptoms, 11-12
Physiologic-motor conditions, 55
Physiotherapy, 99
Poltern, 6
  See also Cluttering
Prejudices, toward stutterers, 43-46
Prevalence, of stuttering, 12
Progressive muscle relaxation, 132,
  133, 172
  See also Relaxation
Protocols, self-control and, 147
Psychic feedback processes, 51
Psychodiagnostic test procedures, 97
Psychological factors, 34, 83
Psychosomatic illness, 65
  drugs and, 134
Psychotherapeutic methods, 99, 100,
  170, 174, 177
  in preventing relapse, 183
Punishment, 60-61, 163
  anxiety and, 107
  in therapy, 106

R

"Rapid therapy program," 125
Reactive pattern, of stutterers, 140
Reading
  as assessment, 75
  speech rhythms in, 103-104
  stuttering confined to, 10
  whispered, 79
  in therapy, 127
  white noise and, 80
Rearing practices, 85
Recordings
  dialogue and, 176-177
  procedure, 129-130
  sound, 127-130
  video, 127-130, 156, 164
Rebounds, 6
Relapse, 181, 183-186
  causes, 184-185

frequency, 179
Relaxation, 169
  See also Progressive muscle
  relaxation
  exercises, 175
  techniques, 132-134, 170-171
Remission
  in children, 162
  spontaneous, 13
Research
  posttherapeutic study, 180-181
  reliability of data, 180
  unsolved problems, 179
Residual air speech, 131
Resistance, of client to therapy, 129
Resocialization, 158-159, 161, 175-176
Rhythmic speech, 63-64, 80, 170, 175
  with children, 165
Role playing, 175
  implementation, 153-154
  in therapy, 151-157
  transfer of skills and, 154-155
  video recordings of, 156

S

Schilling, A.
  age and outcome of therapy, 181
  fear, 141
Schulte, D.
  conditions for behavior, 73
  schema for diagnosis and therapy,
  71
Schulze, C., theory of cognitive
  reconstructions, 127
Schwartz, M. F.
  "blowing technique," 104-105
  laryngospasm, 33
  seven stress-producing stimuli,
  40-41
  sound recordings and therapy,
  130-131
Seeman, M., multidimensional
  therapy, 170, 171
Self-control, 64-65, 126, 137-138,
  139, 146, 175, 184

age and, 162
fear and, 41-42
through speech training, 142-144
stimulus conditions and, 86
successful, 141
techniques developed for, 144-147
in therapy, 140
Self-evaluation, 177
Self-modification, 137, 138, 173-174, 184
motivation for, 146
role playing and, 152
Self-observation, 146-147, 173, 175
in therapy, 175
Self perception, 126
Self-responsibility, attitude, 148
Semantic characteristics, in stutterers, 77-78
Sensory system, and speech sequencing, 56-57
Sentences, therapeutic use, 102
Sentence transposition, 77
Sex differences, 20-21, 27-28, 61-62
delayed auditory feedback and, 114
outcome of therapy and, 181-182
Shadow speech, 29, 64, 110-111, 139, 142
as diversion, 126
Sheehan, J. G.
ambivalence conflicts, 47
conflict and anxiety, 51
role therapy, 175
symptom-stabilizing, 65
"Short therapy," 120
Sign language
as diversion, 126
self-responsibility and, 142
video recordings and, 130
Simultaneous speech, 80, 142
Singing, 11, 63, 64, 165
Situation dependency, 62
Social analysis, 86
Social aspects, 100
Social-cognitive conditions, 55
Social competence, training, 152
Social context, 66-67, 85

Social feedback, 59
Social situations, 92, 94-95, 96
anxiety in, 151
withdrawal from, 149
Social stimuli, 80-81
Social therapy, 157, 172-173
for parents, 171
Speech
aids, 168
gesture language and, 142-143
in avoiding relapse, 183
for self-control, 141-142
use in therapy, 124, 172-176
in transfer of skills, 184
auditory control of, 60
block, 4
breathing and, 6
as communication, 10-11
control, 58
desynchronized coordination, 58-59
development, stutterers vs. nonstutterers, 42-43
difficulties, onset, 56
disfluencies, 7, 11, 59
control of, 41-42
through continuity, 38-39
in normal talkers, 32-33
disordered, 6-7
disturbances, in normal talkers, 27, 58
hearing and, 29-30
fluency, 3, 4
auditory self-control and, 139-140
as cure, 186
establishing, 168
delayed auditory feedback and, 27
as goal of therapy, 100
in stutterers, 59, 64
gestures, as therapy, 103-104
habits, training, 102-103
normal, 5, 31, 39, 59
rhythm, in normal talkers, 103
as therapy, 114-119
self-control, 57, 65

sympton-free, 63
twelve roles of, 101
Spontaneous remission, 62
Stammering (*Stammeln*), 3, 6
clonic stuttering as, 4
stuttering vs., 6, 87-88
Starter, 77, 153
defined, 6
Stier, E., cerebral dominance theory,
23-24
Stop-go mechanism, 77-78
Stress, 40, 65
adaptation and, 9
as cause of stuttering, 44
conditioned tension, 34
-producing stimuli, 40-41
of therapist, 177
unresolvable conflict as, 49
Stutterer
attitude of, 126
labeling, 3
therapist and, 138-139
Stuttering
defined, 3-4
described, 73-74
Symptomatology, 4
in assessment, 75-76
Symptom perception and control,
176
Symptoms
conspicuous, 56
predicting, 125-126
reduction of, 29
therapy and onset, 127

T

Tachyphemia. *See* Cluttering
Terminology, 3
Tessenow, vowel stuttering, 8
"Therapeutic excursions," 157
Therapists
behavior of, 177
and children, 127
Therapy
See also Behavior therapy; Social
therapy

for adults, 166
age-adapted, 171
age differences and, 169, 181
stutterer, 97, 162
attitude toward, 140-141
basic, 169-170
blowing technique, 104-105,
130-131, 132-133, 142
caretakers and, 157-158
combining methods, 161-162, 169
comparison of methods, 179
cure, 186-187
delayed auditory feedback, 30,
112-114, 139, 142
dialogue in, 176-178
differential, 169-170
distinctiveness of methods, 123-124
duration, 182-183
evaluation during, 147
exercises, 143-144
expectations, 187
goals for, 101, 139, 152, 164
groups, 156-157
indications for, 163
individual programs, 100
inhibition, 175
integrative behavior, *171-172*
interdisciplinary decisions, 96
interventions areas, 100
linguistic basis, 77-78
masking, 112
multidimensional, 169, 170
negative practice, 108-110
negligible results, 67
degree of severity and, 180
parents' participation, 163-164
strangers' participation, 157
permanence of results, 176
play, 164-166
posttherapeutic care, 174
preparation for, 167-168
progressive muscle relaxation, 119
reduction of stuttering, 101, 105
repeated, 183, 185-186
requirements, 184-185
role, 175

role playing as, 151-152
self-concept and, 51
self-control and, 137-138, 139
self-modification and, 144-147
sequence for, 166-169
for severe stutterers, 176
sex differences in outcome, 181-182
shadow speech, 110-111
short, 120-122
short-term effects, 123
social, 150
speech aids, 124
    after, 141
for speech disorder only, 67, 150
speech gestures, 103-104
speech rhythm, 114-119
successful, 179
support by caretakers, 158
symptom, 51
transfer to caretaker, 168
Thewall, rhythmic speech, 63-64
Tics, 5
"Time out" procedure, 106-107
Token systems, 106
Tonic stuttering, 4, 15, 75
    negative practice and, 109-110
    remission in, 13
    speech block, 4
    -clonic stuttering, 4
Transfer
    outside of therapy, 150-151,
        154-155, 171, 175, 176, 184-185
    in adults, 166
Treatment. *See* Therapy
Tunner, W.
    biofeedback, 131-132
    environmental vs. constitutional
        factors, 37
    involuntary reflexive qualities, 40
    speech rhythm research, 118
    visual feedback, 106
2 Factor Theory, 42

U

"Unisono method," 170

V

Van Riper, C.
    awareness of client, 126
    children, 12, 15
        speech and hearing, 29
    courses of development, 18-20
    developmental stuttering, 56
    EEGs and stuttering, 23
    environmental factors, 9
    hierarchies in therapy, 151
    integrating procedures, 175
    Jones' hypotheses, 25
    prevalence and extent of
        stuttering, 12
    recoil behavior, 6
    social behavior, 44, 45, 46
Variability, 79
Video feedback, 173
    See also Recordings
Voice exercises, 101
Vowel stuttering, 8

W

Wada test, 24-25
Wendlandt, W.
    caretakers in therapy, 158
    duration of therapy, 182-183
    hierarchies of situations, 151
    resocialization, 158-159, 175-176
Westrich, E.
    fear, 177
    rapport of therapist with client,
        177
Whispering, 165
White noise, 112
    See also Masking
    defined, 28
    delayed auditory feedback and, 28
    as diversion, 126
    reading and, 80
    research using, 31
    speech disturbance and, 59
    stuttering improvement and, 64
    symptom reduction, 29, 30
Word substitution, 77

About the Translator

S. RICHARD SILVERMAN, Ph.D., is Director Emeritus, Central Institute for the Deaf, in St. Louis, Missouri. He is also a Professor Emeritus of audiology at Washington University in St.Louis. He has been a visiting professor and lecturer at numerous American universities as well as schools in India, Pakistan, Latin America, Japan, Australia, Singapore, South Africa, and Israel. Dr. Silverman has served as chairperson, member, and consultant for many professional and governmental organizations that address the problems of the deaf and, upon invitation, has addressed professional and lay groups worldwide about the establishment of audiological facilities and programs. He has published articles in 21 professional journals and coedited one textbook on hearing and deafness and has coauthored one on speech and deafness. Dr. Silverman has received numerous honorary degrees, fellowships, and awards for professional excellence. He has recently been appointed Adjunct Research Scientist at the Institute for Advanced Study of the Communication Processes at the University of Florida, Gainesville, Florida.